Ophthalmic Disease Mechanisms
and Drug Discovery

Ophthalmic Disease Mechanisms and Drug Discovery

Kang Zhang

Editor

Frances Wu

Associate Editor

University of California San Diego

World Scientific

NEW JERSEY · LONDON · SINGAPORE · BEIJING · SHANGHAI · HONG KONG · TAIPEI · CHENNAI · TOKYO

Published by

World Scientific Publishing Co. Pte. Ltd.
5 Toh Tuck Link, Singapore 596224
USA office: 27 Warren Street, Suite 401-402, Hackensack, NJ 07601
UK office: 57 Shelton Street, Covent Garden, London WC2H 9HE

Library of Congress Cataloging-in-Publication Data
Ophthalmic disease mechanisms and drug discovery / [edited by] Kang Zhang.
　　p. ; cm.
　Includes bibliographical references and index.
　ISBN 978-9814663069 (hardcover : alk. paper)
　I. Zhang, Kang, editor.
　[DNLM: 1. Eye Diseases--drug therapy. 2. Drug Discovery--methods.
3. Eye Diseases--diagnosis. 4. Eye Diseases--physiopathology. WW 166]
　RE994
　617.7'061--dc23
                                    2015032208

British Library Cataloguing-in-Publication Data
A catalogue record for this book is available from the British Library.

Typeset by Stallion Press
Email: enquiries@stallionpress.com

Contents

Introduction

Kang Zhang

Progress in the fields of molecular biology and genomics has significantly improved our knowledge of ocular disorders and their pathogenesis in recent decades. Technological advances in ophthalmic imaging have allowed us to more thoroughly characterize these diseases clinically and monitor their progression over time. Such efforts have resulted in viable therapeutic targets for disorders previously considered untreatable. In particular, the advent of anti-angiogenic therapy has led to improved outcomes for many people afflicted with sight-threatening neovascular diseases. It is therefore of crucial importance for clinicians and scientists to stay up-to-date on the latest information.

This book provides a concise summary of several major topics in ophthalmology, and also highlights a variety of new therapeutic paradigms currently under investigation. Nanotechnology represents one such promising approach. With the use of nanoparticles, it addresses challenges associated with drug delivery to the posterior segment of the eye. In addition, exciting novel developments in pharmacogenomics are playing an increasingly greater role in our understanding and treatment of ophthalmic diseases. Pharmacogenomics paves the way for more individualized therapy tailored to patients' unique genetic backgrounds.

The information contained in this book will be useful to researchers, practicing ophthalmologists, fellows, and residents. It is intended to describe recent advancements in the genetics and molecular mechanisms of ophthalmic diseases, with an emphasis on novel treatment strategies and future directions for drug discovery.

1

Chapter 1: Pathology and Mechanism of Eye Diseases

Katherine J. Wert[†], Heike Kroeger[‡], Frances Wu[‡],
*Stephen H. Tsang[§], and Jonathan H. Lin[‡,**]*

[†]*The Whitehead Institute for Biomedical Research,*
Cambridge, MA 02142

[‡]*Departments of Pathology and Ophthalmology,*
University of California San Diego, La Jolla, CA 92093

[§]*Departments of Ophthalmology, Pathology, and Cell Biology,*
Columbia University College of Physicians and Surgeons,
New York, NY 10032

[**]*VA San Diego Healthcare System, San Diego, CA 92161*

1. Introduction

Retinal degenerative diseases are the leading cause of irreversible blindness in Western nations, and the loss of sight affects over 3.4 million people in the United States alone.[1] These diseases have high genetic and allelic heterogeneity, and therefore our understanding of the pathophysiology of these conditions is limited. However, progress in molecular genetics has determined specific factors that play significant roles in the pathogenesis of retinal degeneration. This chapter is focused on understanding the pathology of the human eye, the molecular genetics identified in degenerative diseases of the eye, and the current known mechanisms for these diseases.

2. The Eye

The human eye is a complex organ that consists of many different cell types. The eye transmits information to be processed by the brain on the color, form, and light intensity of objects. The human eye can be divided into two main parts: the anterior and the posterior segments.[2]

2.1. Anterior eye

In the anterior portion, the sclera and cornea act as outer protective layers of the eye. Also anterior in the eye is the uveal tract, composed of the iris, ciliary body, and anterior choroid. The components of the uveal tract mainly function under the control of the autonomic nervous system. The uveal tract allows for the exchange of nutrition and gases into the posterior portion of the eye. The ciliary body and the iris are directly supplied by the uveal vessels, while these vessels indirectly support the sclera, lens, and outer retina via diffusible nutrients. The uveal tract contains numerous melanocytes that reduce the light reflected within the eye and absorb light transmitted through the sclera, in order to improve the retinal image.[2] Moreover, the ciliary body produces an aqueous humor and regulates the contour of the translucent lens, thereby controlling the focus of the eye. The iris provides the eye pigmentation, as well as pupil dilation and constriction to allow for varying levels of retinal illumination. The choroid is a vascular layer that supplies the outer retina and the retinal pigment epithelium (RPE), both parts of the posterior eye as described in the next section.

2.2. Posterior eye

The posterior eye consists of the RPE and the neurosensory retina.[3,4] The RPE creates a selective permeability barrier between the outer choriocapillaris vasculature of the eye and the inner sensory retina, and this is known as the outer blood-retinal barrier.[4] It is comprised of a pigmented monolayer of RPE cells. The RPE monolayer consists of cells cuboidal in shape in the periphery of the eye, to columnar in shape nearing the macular region of the eye. The barrier function of the RPE allows for the provision of nutrients, such as vitamin A metabolites, as well as the clearing of photoreceptor outer segment (POS) debris daily from the overlying photoreceptor cell layer.[5–9] Between each RPE cell there are tight junctions and ion transporters, which create electrical potential differences between the apical and basal surfaces of the cell as well as intercellular communications. Using this electrical potential, the RPE cells regulate the composition, such as pH, of the photoreceptor extracellular matrix and protect the visual function of the retina. Additionally, the RPE cells contain microvilli on the apical surface, which help phagocytose the POS debris as well as transport enzymes from the basal to apical surface to contact the inner retinal layers.

2.2.1. The retina

The retina is composed of different types of neurons that each form distinct synapses with one another.[4] The retina transduces the optical properties of an image into neural signals, which are then transmitted through the retinal cell layers to the visual cortex of the brain. The outermost layer of neurons, overlying the RPE monolayer, is the photoreceptor cell layer. These photoreceptor cells create a mosaic pattern of light and darkness that reflect the optical properties of the image, which cause repetitive discharges to the bipolar cells. The bipolar cells then synapse to the ganglion cells, whose axons comprise the nerve fiber layer and the optic nerve. The ganglion cells then discharge the mosaic pattern of light and darkness to the brain, to comprise the visual image.

In addition to these three cell types, there are the horizontal, amacrine, and Müller glial cells. The horizontal cells synapse with the bipolar neurons and photoreceptor cells, while the amacrine cells synapse between the bipolar cells and the ganglion cells. The Müller glial cells span the width of the entire retina, from the inner limiting membrane to the outer limiting membrane where the Müller glial cells form junctions with the photoreceptor cells. The complex neurocircuitry of the retina relies on the signaling mosaicism of the light-sensitive photoreceptor cells, as will be described further in the next sections.

2.2.2. The photoreceptor cells

The photoreceptor cells are the light-sensing neurons directly overlying the RPE. There are two types of photoreceptor cells in the retina: the rods and the cones. The majority of the photoreceptor cells, approximately 97%, are comprised of the rods, while the remaining 3% consist of the cones. Both the rod and cone photoreceptor cells have specific roles for the amount and type of light required for their signaling synaptic response. The rod cells respond to single photons of light, and are therefore highly sensitive and react in low-light, nighttime visual settings. The rod cells have a response of up to 10,000 photons per second, known as mesopic vision, a response range of three orders of magnitude before saturation.[10] At the point of rod cell saturation, the cone cells begin to sense photons of light. The cone cells act as photopic vision, responding up to 10 billion photons per second and providing daytime sight for the human eye. In addition, there are three forms of cone cells in the human eye, the S-, M-, and L-cones, which respond to specific wavelengths of light and provide for color vision.

The human eye is enriched in specific regions for each of these photoreceptor cell types, which provide the visual signals that are sensed daily in an individual's life. The central region of the retina, known as the macula, is enriched with cone cells. This allows for bright light and color vision in the central visual field, while the rod photoreceptor cells enrich the peripheral visual field.[10,11] Of note, pathological diseases affecting vision will either cause a loss of function of the rod or the cone photoreceptor cells, or both. Depending on which cell type is affected, the patient will exhibit a loss of nighttime vision and the peripheral visual field (rod cell loss-of-function) or a loss of color vision and the central visual field (cone cell loss-of-function).

Both the rod and cone photoreceptor cells each consist of an outer segment, an inner segment, a cell body, and a synaptic terminal that allows for their transmission to the second-order neurons of the retina. The inner segment of the photoreceptor cells contains the mitochondria, ribosomes, endoplasmic reticulum, Golgi, and vesicles that assemble and transport opsin molecules to the outer segment discs for the visual cycle and phototransduction cascade.[12] In the rods, the outer segment has detached stacks of disc structures, formed by invaginations of the plasma membrane at its base.[12] In contrast, the cones consist of discs that remain attached to the outer segment membrane. For both cell types, the outer segments are being continuously produced and shed during the mammalian circadian rhythm. For the rod cells, the outer segment turnover occurs in the morning, while the outer segment turnover of the cone cells occurs in the evening. The RPE apical microvilli envelop the outer segments and separate the most distal discs from the remaining outer segment stacks. These "shed" discs are phagocytosed and degraded by the RPE, allowing for the constant turnover of the outer segments and the stable length of the outer segments within the retina.[12–14] These outer segments comprise part of the neurocircuitry required for visual processing, which occurs from the photoreceptor cells to the ganglion cells and optic nerve.

3. The Phototranduction Cascade

The multiple cell layers of the neurosensory retina are important for the visual cycle and phototransduction. In pathological disease states, these cell layers become disrupted and disorganized. In normal states, photons pass through the anterior eye and the retinal cell layers and are absorbed by the RPE. The photon of light causes a conformational change in the visual pigment, rhodopsin (RHO), which then activates a signaling cascade that leads to a ganglion cell action potential in the optic nerve. This action potential relays from the optic nerve to the lateral geniculate nucleus and other centers, such as the suprachiasmatic nucleus and visual cortex of the brain. The process in which energy from light is absorbed and translated into an electrical impulse sent to the central nervous system is known as the phototransduction cascade.

In the dark, RHO is not activated. A molecule called transducin (Gt$\alpha\beta\gamma$) is bound together in its heterotrimeric form, and another molecule called cGMP phosphodiesterase 6 (PDE6) is in its PDE6$\alpha\beta\gamma$ inactive form. As a result, there is high cytoplasmic cGMP, and the cGMP-gated Na$^+$/Ca^{2+} ion (CNG) channels in the plasma membrane of the photoreceptor cell remain open. This allows for a circulating current within the photoreceptor cell. This circulating current releases glutamate from the synaptic terminal in the outer plexiform layer, signaling to the second-order neurons of the retina. When photons of light are sensed by the photoreceptor cell, the current in the outer segment is interrupted through a cascade known as phototransduction.[15] The phototransduction cascade is carefully regulated by key molecules involved in the activation, deactivation, and adaptation of the cascade within the photoreceptor cell.

3.1. Activation of the phototransduction cascade

The visual cycle leads to the formation of 11-*cis*-retinal in the RPE, which is shuttled into the outer segment of the photoreceptor cell to non-covalently bind opsin and make RHO. Photons of light are sensed in the photoreceptor cell outer segment, activating and causing a conformational change in RHO to form metarhodopsin II (Rh*). Rh* activates Gtαβγ, which is located in the outer segment. Gtαβγ molecules are heterotrimeric G-proteins that contain alpha (Gtα), beta (Gtβ), and gamma (Gtγ) subunits. Gtαβγ exchanges guanosine diphosphate (GDP) for guanosine triphosphate (GTP) within the photoreceptor cell.[16] The activation of Gtαβγ by Rh* causes GTP to bind to the Gta subunit. This Gtα-GTP complex dissociates from Gtαβγ and binds to two inhibitory subunits on PDE6.[17]

PDE6 is the primary regulator of cytoplasmic cGMP concentration in photoreceptor cells, and plays a highly important role in the phototransduction cascade. It has slightly different forms in rod versus cone cells. In the rod cell, PDE6 is a heterotetrameric protein that contains a catalytic α-subunit, a catalytic β-subunit, and two inhibitory γ-subunits. In contrast, PDE6 contains a catalytic dimer of two identical α′-subunits in the cone cell, rather than the α- and β-subunits found in the rod photoreceptor. Furthermore, the size and composition of the γ′-inhibitory subunits in the cone cell differ from that of the rod cell γ-inhibitory PDE6 subunits.[18] However, the overall response to light stimulation remains similar for both rods and cones. The binding of Gtα-GTP on the inhibitory γ-subunits of PDE6 removes the inhibition and allows for the catalytic activity of the α- and β-subunits.[16,17,19] The catalytically active PDE6αβ hydrolyzes cGMP at a rapid rate, reducing its concentration in the photoreceptor cell cytoplasm and shutting down the CNG channels.[20] The closing of the CNG channels halts the influx of Na^+ and Ca^{2+}, reducing their levels within the photoreceptor cell and causing the cell to become hyperpolarized. Hyperpolarization of the photoreceptor decreases glutamate release from its synaptic terminal to the bipolar and ganglion cells of the retina.

3.2. Deactivation of the phototransduction cascade

The phototransduction cascade undergoes deactivation after light stimulation, in order to return cGMP to basal levels. To get to this point, the photo-excited Rh* is phosphorylated at the threonine and serine residues at its carboxyl tail by RHO-specific G-protein-dependent receptor kinase I (GRK1).[12] The reduction in Ca^{2+} levels after closure of the CNG channels reduces inhibition on GRK1 by a molecule called Recoverin. The phosphorylated Rh* (Rh*-P) is inactivated, and binds to Arrestin (Arr; also called S-antigen) more efficiently than Gtα. Arr removes the phosphate groups from Rh*, and thus rapidly reduces the dephosphorylated, active Rh* that is available for the continuing activation of Gtα in the phototransduction cascade.[21] Alongside the inactivation of Rh*, Gtα has intrinsic GTPase activity and therefore inactivates itself after it binds to the inhibitory subunits of PDE6.[22] This process is accelerated by the presence of a membrane-associated protein known as the regulator of G-protein signaling (RGS9).[23] The removal of Gtα from the PDE6 γ-inhibitory subunits allows for them to re-associate with the α- and β-subunits to inactivate the complex. At the same time, two retinal guanylate cyclases, Ret GC-1 and Ret GC-2, are activated by the loss of intracellular Ca^{2+}, and catalyze cGMP synthesis in the photoreceptor cell.[12] This activation occurs via guanylate cyclase-activating proteins, known as GCAP-1/p-20 and GCAP-2/p-24.[24–26] Once cGMP returns to basal concentrations, the CNG channels in the plasma membrane re-open and the deactivation of the phototransduction cascade is complete. It is important to note that the cascade can be re-activated rapidly when Rh*-P-Arr associates with 11-*cis*-retinal. This leads to the dissociation of Arr, and phosphatase 2A can bind and dephosphorylate Rh*-P to return it to its activated form. This process continues until the photoreceptor adapts to constant light stimulation.

3.3. Adaptation of the phototransduction cascade

Prolonged exposure to light leads to an adaptation of the photoreceptor cell to the light stimulation. First, Recoverin's inhibition of GRK1 is reduced during prolonged light exposure, allowing for GRK1 to increase its activity. Secondly, Ca^{2+}-sensitive members of the protein kinase C family phosphorylate the released γ-inhibitory subunits of PDE6 at threonine 35 during light stimulation. This causes a more rapid binding of the inhibitory subunits to the PDE6αβ complex for inhibition of PDE6 catalytic activity on cGMP. Lastly, the CNG channel is bound to a molecule called calmodulin at high Ca^{2+} concentrations, and with prolonged light exposure the calmodulin is released and the CNG channel affinity for cGMP is reduced.[27] This results in the CNG channels opening at a lower level of cGMP than under normal dark conditions.

4. The Visual Cycle

The visual cycle is the system that provides the 11-*cis* retinal chromophore for phototransduction. The outer segment disc contains several million opsin molecules, which are non-covalently bonded to 11-*cis* retinal, a vitamin A derivative, in the dark. This opsin bonded to 11-*cis*-retinal creates the visual pigment known as RHO.[28] RHO is a seven-loop transmembrane G-protein-coupled receptor that has a protonated Schiff base with a lysine side chain. This lysine side chain links to the 11-*cis* retinal chromophore.[18,29] Photon absorption causes the isomerization of 11-*cis* retinal to all-*trans* retinal, which dissociates from opsin in the outer segment membrane. Phosphatidylethanolamine binds the all-*trans* retinal and forms *N*-retinylidene-phosphatidylethanolamine, which is transported into the cytosol by an ATP-binding cassette transporter (ABCA4; also known as Rim protein). In the cytosol of the photoreceptor cell, all-*trans* retinal is reduced by retinal dehydrogenase to vitamin A (all-*trans* retinol), which is transported out of the photoreceptor cell and into the RPE. In the RPE, lecithin-retinol acyltransferase (LRAT) esterifies the all-*trans* retinol, it is then isomerized by retinal pigment epithelial 65-kDa (RPE65) to 11-*cis* retinol, and 11-*cis* retinol dehydrogenase (RDH5) oxidizes it into 11-*cis* retinal. The 11-*cis* retinal is then transported from the RPE back into the photoreceptor via the interphotoreceptor retinoid binding protein (IRBP), and can bind to opsin to form another molecule of RHO.[30]

5. Pathology of Eye Diseases

Mutations within the proteins responsible for the renewal and shedding of photoreceptor outer segments, visual transduction, and retinol metabolism, among others, have a great impact on the health of retinal cells and the ability to signal accurate electrical impulses to the brain for image formation. The majority of retinal degenerative diseases are caused by genetic defects that lead to reduced protein levels or incorrect protein functions.[5,12,31]

5.1. *Leber congenital amaurosis*

Leber congenital amaurosis (LCA) is the most common inherited cause of early-onset visual impairment, and is primarily associated with mutations in RPE65.[32] LCA patients present during infancy or early childhood with night blindness, a tendency to fixate on bright light sources, and moderate to severe visual limitations. White dots and granules are visible in the RPE of young children, and visual acuity drops from approximately 6/30–6/190 in early childhood to 3/360 by 18 years of age. Upon fundus examination in later years, retinal atrophy and attenuation of the retinal vasculature are noticeable. Electroretinograms (ERGs) display a loss of rod and cone cell function.[33] Currently, there is one identified gene that causes an autosomal dominant form of LCA, and 11 identified genes for autosomal recessive forms of the disease, although more genes are mapped for potentially playing a role.[34]

5.2. *Retinitis pigmentosa*

Aside from LCA, the majority of genetic mutations in the phototransduction cascade are linked to autosomal dominant (adRP) and autosomal recessive (arRP) forms of retinitis pigmentosa, or RP-related conditions. RP is the most common cause of hereditary blindness worldwide, affecting more than 1:3000 people, and can be classified into four patterns of inheritance: adRP (15–20% of cases), arRP (20–25% of cases), X-linked RP (10–15% of cases), and mitochondrial RP. For the remaining 40–55% of unclassified cases, the patients have no known family history of RP, and the disease is considered to be simplex RP although most are believed to be arRP.[35,36] adRP is usually a late-onset disease, with mild phenotypes, while arRP is more severe and typically presents during the first decade of life.[37] There are also syndromic forms of RP, where the disease presents with over 30 systemic abnormalities as seen in Usher syndrome (associated with deafness) and Bardet-Biedl syndrome (associated variably with obesity, polydactyly, mental retardation, and infertility), as will be discussed later in the chapter.[36]

Individuals with RP present with nyctalopia (night blindness), which progresses to tunnel vision (constricted visual field due to the loss of rod photoreceptor cells). The central vision, important for reading and facial recognition, remains relatively normal until the secondary death of cone cells at a later stage of disease. In some patients, cystoid macular edema will lead to an earlier loss of the central visual field. Although there is disease heterogeneity, the majority of patients will exhibit grayish discoloration of the RPE upon fundus examination, known as bone spicules. This is associated with intraretinal pigment migration from the outer to inner retina, coalescing around the blood vessels. In addition, optic disc drusen, macular edema, posterior subscapular cataracts, and vitreous cells are frequently reported. As the disease progresses, significant attenuation of the retinal vasculature occurs, and the optic nerve develops a "waxy" pallor. Full field ERGs display a loss of the rod-specific b-wave amplitude consistent with rod cell dysfunction, as well as a reduction in the rod-driven maximal a-wave amplitude, without the presence of cone cell dysfunction as seen by a normal 30-Hz flicker response.[38,39]

6. Mechanisms of Eye Diseases

RP is an important model for studying neurodegenerative diseases, mainly because the pathogenic disease progression in RP can be generalized to that of other retinal degenerations, such as age-related macular degeneration (AMD) and LCA. There are a number of genes within the visual cycle and phototransduction cascade that have been linked to arRP, such as *ABCA4*, *RPE65*, and *LRAT*. Many of these same genes show phenotypic heterogeneity, as they have also been associated with other progressive and stationary retinal diseases. For example, mutations in *RPE65* have been identified for LCA and nystagmus, while mutations in *ABCA4* are identified for Stargardt macular dystrophy and cone-rod dystrophy, with correlation to AMD.[1,40–42]

Retinal diseases are classified according to the clinical history, fundus examination, electrophysiological studies, and psychophysical studies. Their true classifications, however, remain ambiguous, as many retinal degenerative diseases arising from different genetic mechanisms can present similarly. For example, RP can be caused by mutations in the phototransduction cascade (RHO or PDE6) as well as by mutations in rod outer segment proteins such as peripherin.[43,44] Conversely, mutations within the same locus may demonstrate phenotypic variability; for example, mutations in PDE6β can cause both RP and congenital stationary night blindness. It is currently unknown how one mutation can lead to a progressive, degenerative disease such as RP, while a different mutation affecting the same locus will result in non-progressive visual dysfunction.

What is currently known is that each of the genes involved in retinal degenerative diseases functions in various ways, coding for proteins involved in phototransduction, structural support, intracellular transport, transcription, or splicing. Each of these mechanisms will be discussed in the next section. Although the basic mechanisms that lead to rod cell death, and secondarily cone cell death, in RP are not well characterized, the study of this degenerative disease has greatly contributed to the characterization of metabolic and biochemical pathways in photoreceptor cells.

6.1. *Rod photoreceptor cell metabolism*

Rod photoreceptor cells have specific metabolic needs that vary whether there is light saturation or dark adaptation. In the light, there is an increase in anabolic activity of the rod cell, during which time the outer segments are both shed and renewed.[45] There is a reduction in oxidative phosphorylation, as the rod cell consumption of oxygen (O_2) is shown to be reduced by more than 30% in both macaques and cat model systems.[46–48] In the dark, however, the rod photoreceptors switch their metabolic needs to be able to consume large quantities of adenosine triphosphate (ATP). ATP consumption is required for the functioning of the ion transporters, as one ATP is consumed each time Ca^{2+} is exported and each time three Na^+ ions are exported.[49] Therefore, rod cells utilize both glycolysis and oxidative phosphorylation in the dark to meet this metabolic need.[45,50] However, the mechanism by which rod photoreceptors switch from glycolysis (in the dark) to anabolic activity (in the light) is largely unknown.

Recently, the hypoxic retina has become an area of interest concerning rod cell death in various retinal degenerative diseases. For instance, the early pathology seen in AMD patients is the deposition of subretinal drusen and the thickening of Bruch's membrane.[51] This leads to retinal ischemia, since there is a decrease in O_2 diffusion between the choriocapillaris and the RPE. Another early pathological feature of AMD is the loss of dark adaptation, suggesting that rod photoreceptor cell function has declined in these patients.[52] It is possible that hypoxia and retinal ischemia are key mechanisms by which macular degeneration occurs in AMD.

Hypoxia inducible factor 1 (HIF1) is upregulated in hypoxic conditions and activates the transcription of certain genes, many of which are involved in the promotion of glycolysis and the inhibition of the tricarboxylic acid (TCA) cycle.[53,54] HIF1 is known to be upregulated in patients with diabetic retinopathy (DR) and has been implicated as a potential target in cancer therapies, as it has been shown to drive anaerobic glycolysis and regulate cancer metabolism.[55,56] Furthermore cancer research has shown that SIRT6 acts as a tumor suppressor, and may play an opposing role to HIF1 in retinal degeneration. Another member of the sirtuin family, SIRT1, has recently been shown to inhibit HIF1 and VEGF signaling, providing a potential regulatory effect of the sirtuin family proteins in rod photoreceptor metabolism.[57] However, it remains uncertain whether there is a specific mechanism of rod cell metabolism and oxidative phosphorylation that leads to rod degeneration, and the specific roles of HIF1 and the sirtuin family still need to be explored.

6.2. The complement pathway and the alternative pathway

In addition to HIF1 and the sirtuin family of proteins, hypoxia has been shown to play a role in various retinal degenerative diseases, such as AMD and DR. Recent studies have shown that retinal hypoxia leads to upregulation of the alternative pathway via complement factor B.[58] The complement pathway is vital in providing an immune response against foreign pathogens and maintaining immune system homeostasis. There are three pathways that regulate this process: the classical complement pathway, the alternative pathway, and the lecithin pathway. The inhibition of the alternative pathway in knockout mouse models protected photoreceptor cells from death during retinal detachment, suggesting a key role for this pathway in the mechanism of photoreceptor death during hypoxia.

Furthermore, other studies have implicated the alternative pathway in AMD pathogenesis.[59] Complement factor H (CFH), a component of the complement pathway that binds to host cell surfaces via glycosaminoglycans, allows for the system to correctly identify foreign pathogens without damaging host tissue. CFH is a known inhibitor of the alternative pathway, and it has recently been determined that decreasing CFH induces the formation of sub-RPE deposits.[60] These sub-RPE deposits are believed to activate the complement pathway, contributing to RPE damage and the impairment of visual function. However, the precise mechanisms by which the complement pathway and the alternative pathway act during photoreceptor degeneration remain unknown.

6.3. Lipofuscin accumulation

The accumulation of lipofuscin provides another mechanism by which RPE deposits are involved in retinal degenerative diseases. Lipofuscin is composed of *N*-retinylidene-*N*-retinylethanolamine (A2E), which is formed by the combination of *N*-retinylidene-phosphatidylethanolamine with all-*trans* retinaldehyde. Lipofuscin accumulation is a clinical feature of Stargardt macular dystrophy, AMD, some forms of RP, and other retinal dystrophic diseases.[61] It is thought to be caused by dysfunction of the Rim protein, allowing for *N*-retinylidene-phosphatidylethanolamine to build up in outer segment discs that are then phagocytosed by the RPE. This is supported by evidence that the varying severities of disease in AMD patients appear to be associated with the level of functional Rim protein still present in the retina.[62] Although the exact mechanism of cell death via lipofuscin is not fully elucidated, A2E is believed to be toxic to the RPE cells. It is thought that A2E within the RPE causes toxicity by increasing membrane permeability, leading to lysosomal dysfunction in the monolayer, and detaching pro-apoptotic proteins that initiate a cell-death pathway within the cell.[63–68]

6.4. *Non-autonomous cone cell death*

One very well established mechanism in RP is the death of rod photore-ceptor cells that is a direct consequence of the disease mutation. However, the loss of cone photoreceptor cells as the disease progresses is second-ary to the loss of the rod cells, and therefore non-cell autonomous. Since cone cells comprise only 3% of the photoreceptors, with rods making up the remaining 97% of photoreceptor cells, it is highly likely that the sec-ondary cone cell death is caused by the loss of rod photoreceptor cells. However, the pathophysiology underlying this secondary loss of cone cells remains unknown. It is thought that cone cell death arises from both a decrease in survival factors produced by healthy rod cells during dis-ease progression and an increase in toxic factors secreted by the diseased and dying rod photoreceptors.

6.5. *Calcium-dependent apoptosis*

The precise mechanisms causing rod cell death are unclear; however, it is believed that the constitutive activation of the phototransduction cascade support a Ca^{2+}-dependent apoptotic pathway.[69] The *Pde6βrd1* mouse model, carrying a mutation in the beta subunit of PDE6, provides evidence that loss of PDE6 activity contributes to defects in the outer segment of the photoreceptor cell, the accumulation of cGMP within the photoreceptor, and likely the accumulation of excess intracellular Ca^{2+}.[18,29,70] Since intra-cellular Ca^{2+} is highly regulated, the variation in Ca^{2+} levels may initiate an apoptotic response.[71] The same process is thought to occur in other retinal degenerative mutations, such as in *RPE65*. In these cases, the loss-of-function of the diseased protein leads to continual activation of the pho-totransduction cascade via RHO noise levels, a theory known as the "equivalent light hypothesis."[69,71–74] The phototransduction cascade remains constitutively active via an unbound opsin-generated signal to guanine nucleotide binding protein alpha transducing activity polypeptide 1 (GNAT1). In mammalian models carrying this mutation, such as the *Rpe65tm1/Rpe65tm1* mouse model, the cascade is active independent of light or dark conditions. Thus, this mutation causes a decline in intracel-lular Ca^{2+} levels that can trigger an apoptotic pathway.

Ca^{2+} ions regulate apoptosis through at least four known systems: Ca^{2+}-activated phosphatases (e.g. calcineurin), type II and type IV Ca^{2+}/calmodulin-depended protein kinases (CaMK), Ca^{2+}-dependent protein kinase C (PKC), and Ca^{2+}-sensitive adenylate cyclases. One reason the Ca^{2+}-dependent apoptotic pathway is implicated in retinal degeneration is that the activation of calcineurin by Ca^{2+} dephosphorylates the Bcl-2-associated death promoter (Bad). This causes Bad to dissociate from its complex in the cytosol and migrate into the mitochondria, where it dimerizes with Bcl-2 family members such as Bcl-xL and promotes apoptosis.[75]

6.6. *The unfolded protein response*

Additionally, the cGMP and Ca^{2+} cation concentrations within the photoreceptor cell may interfere with the formation of new outer segment discs, leading to the death of the photoreceptor, or they may initiate the unfolded protein response (UPR), which would lead to apoptosis. The UPR is an important regulatory mechanism of the endoplasmic reticulum (ER), which is a membranous organelle network responsible for protein folding and maturation of membrane and secretory proteins; free intracellular calcium storage; and lipid/sterol synthesis. Impairment of protein folding and other ER functions can cause ER stress.[76] Prolonged and uncontrolled ER stress ultimately leads to cell death.[77] A growing number of studies have demonstrated the role of ER stress in many retinal dystrophies caused by genetic mutations that lead to protein misfolding.[5,78] For example, the P23H RHO mutation, which is the most common cause of heritable RP in the North American population, as well as the T17M RHO and S334ter RHO mutations, have all been shown to have ER stress as a hallmark of the disease.[79–85] ER stress is also found in retinal degeneration models that do not involve protein misfolding events, such as light- and dark-induced changes or increased intracellular calcium levels in photoreceptors, as witnessed for the retinal degeneration 1 (rd1) mouse strain.[86–89]

One retinal dystrophic disease known to be caused by ER stress and the UPR is the autosomal recessive disorder achromatopsia (ACHM). ACHM is characterized by a loss of visual acuity, nystagmus, color blindness, and photophobia. Activating transcription factor 6 (ATF6) is a 90-kDa transmembrane transcription factor that regulates ER stress and the homeostasis of the ER. Mutations in the *ATF6* gene have been shown to cause ACHM in human patients as well as in murine model systems.[90] *Atf6-/-* mutant mice are unable to activate the adaptive UPR transcriptional response to ER stress, suggesting that ATF6 function is required for activation of the UPR and photoreceptor cell survival in the presence of ER stress.

One of the interesting questions that remains is: how does misfolded rhodopsin actually cause photoreceptor cell death? UPR signaling seems to play a very important role in the induction of photoreceptor cell death. UPR signaling is mediated by a group of intracellular signal transduction pathways that detect protein misfolding in the ER and transmit that information to the rest of the cell to facilitate protective or pro-apoptotic actions. Under acute ER stress, UPR signaling can increase the amount of ER membrane in order to facilitate its growth. UPR upregulates ER-resident chaperones and protein-modifying enzymes in an attempt to help the cell cope with the abnormal accumulation of misfolded proteins and to restore ER homeostasis. If ER stress persists, the UPR triggers apoptosis.[76,91]

Multiple animal models of retinal degeneration have identified the UPR signaling pathways as abnormally activated in a temporal manner that correlates with the death of photoreceptor cells in the retina.[83,85,92,93] These findings raise the intriguing possibility that UPR signaling presents a molecular link between rhodopsin misfolding in the ER of photoreceptors and the induction of apoptosis, which ultimately leads to photoreceptor cell death and blindness.

Recently, it was shown that after activating the protective branch of the UPR signaling pathway, mutant P23H RHO is efficiently degraded from the rod cell using the proteasomal ER-associated protein degradation machinery (ERAD).[94,95] It was further demonstrated that the loss of RHO protein occurred as soon as photoreceptors developed, therefore preceding photoreceptor cell death. This finding reveals that one of the earliest and significant pathophysiological effects of ER stress and UPR signaling in photoreceptors is the highly efficient elimination of misfolded RHO protein. Disruption of protein homeostasis in photoreceptor cells may be a common factor in retinal degeneration.[94-96] However, further experiments are required to identify the precise mechanism of photoreceptor cell death.

6.7. Ciliary defects

The photoreceptor cell contains a primary cilium that bridges the inner and outer segments, to transfer the structural and protein synthesis machinery into the outer segment for phototransduction. Since there is a daily turnover of outer segment discs in the photoreceptors, the continual trafficking of these important proteins by the primary cilium is necessary for photoreceptor function and structural morphology. Ciliary defects are thought to be responsible for many retinal degenerative diseases, such as LCA and systemic RP disorders.

Bardet-Biedl syndrome (BBS) is a cone-rod dystrophic disease with systemic abnormalities such as polydactyly, obesity, renal malformations, gonadal malformations, and learning disabilities. BBS patients typically become legally blind in the second decade of life, and present with macular and optic disc atrophy, pigmentary changes, and a loss of ERG response for both rod and cone photoreceptor cells. BBS genes have been identified, and some of these genes are involved in retrograde protein trafficking (*BBS3* and *BBS6*) and anchoring of the microtubule for transport of proteins (*BBS8*).[97–99] There is a knockout BBS2 mouse model, and these mice reflect the human BBS condition by sharing phenotypes such as retinopathy, renal cysts, impaired olfaction and spermatogenesis, and obesity.[100] Interestingly, the UPR was recently found to be activated in BBS animal models, and pharmacologic modulation of UPR partially improved retinal function in these mice, suggesting that UPR signaling may be linked to ciliary defects in BBS.[101]

Another systemic RP-related disorder is Usher syndrome, which is the most common form of syndromic RP and causes 20–40% of arRP cases. Clinical presentation of Usher syndrome is divided into three types: Type I, Type II, and Type III. Type I Usher syndrome is the most severe, with patients having congenital deafness, vision impairment and vestibular dysfunction in the first few decades of life. Type II and Type III Usher syndrome occur later in life with symptoms similar to other arRP patients. Proteins that are identified to be involved in Usher syndrome include motor proteins (myosin VIIa), adhesion molecules, G-protein coupled receptors (GPR98/VLGR1b), and signaling proteins (harmonin).[97] It is believed that proteins leading to Usher syndrome are localized to the primary cilium and involved in protein scaffolding for the bridging of microtubules in the photoreceptor cell, as well as with its synaptic signaling pathways.

Furthermore, mutations in RP GTPase regulator interacting protein (RPGR-IP) and centrosomal protein 290-kDa (CEP290), two proteins in complex with one another, are associated with both LCA and X-linked RP.[102–105] RPGR-IP links the primary cilium of the photoreceptor to RPGR, and loss-of-function of this protein causes abnormal outer segment disc morphogenesis and the mislocalization of structural and phototransduction-related proteins within the photoreceptor cell.[106] In addition, RPGR mutations lead to intracellular trafficking defects within the photoreceptor cell, a mechanism common to many retinal degenerative diseases.

6.8. *Intracellular trafficking defects*

A prime example of a disease with intracellular trafficking defects is choroideremia. Choroideremia is an X-linked retinal degenerative disease that causes night blindness in early adulthood and a loss of central acuity and the visual field in the fifth and sixth decades of life. Fundus examination of patients with choroideremia displays large scalloped areas of RPE and choriocapillaris atrophy, beginning at the periphery and developing centrally over time until macular atrophy is visible. Some carriers of choroideremia, although asymptomatic, may show changes upon ERG examination and visible fundus abnormalities.

Choroideremia is caused by a mutation in Rab escort protein 1 (REP1). REP1 assists geranylgeranyl transferase to add geranyl groups to the Rab escort protein.[107] Rab escort protein is responsible for the movement of organelles, such as lysosomes, vesicles, and endosomes, and the geranyl groups are necessary to link Rab protein to the compartment membranes for movement and function. The mechanism by which REP1 mutations cause cell degeneration in choroideremia patients is debated. Zebrafish studies have suggested a primary role of the RPE, where REP1 mutations cause defects in the RPE ability to phagocytose photoreceptor outer segments, creating RPE degeneration that leads to secondary loss of the photoreceptors and choriocapillaris.[108,109] Mechanisms directly causing photoreceptor cell degeneration are unknown; however, it is clear that defects in intracellular trafficking play a role in vision loss.

6.9. Structural defects

Both adRP and arRP, along with other retinal degenerative diseases, may be caused by mutations in proteins that provide the structural scaffolding of the photoreceptor cell. Mutations in the retinal degeneration slow (*RDS*) gene leads to approximately 5% of adRP cases. The *RDS* gene is known to encode a 39-kDa glycoprotein, peripherin.[110] Peripherin is a member of the tetraspanin family of proteins, containing four transmembrane domains that localize it to the rim of the photoreceptor outer segment discs. The protein is believed to scaffold the outer segment discs to the cytoskeleton, although there is no direct evidence. Loss-of-function of peripherin in a mouse model results in a lack of photoreceptor outer segments and subsequent slow degeneration of the photoreceptor cells.[111–113] In humans, *RDS* mutations have highly variable phenotypes that do not match the mouse model system, even with the same specific gene mutation.[110] Therefore, environmental interactions or other modifiers may affect the phenotypic outcome of the disease.

The Crumbs protein complex has been identified to play a role in arRP disease. There are three Crumbs protein homologs found in humans: CRB1 (localized to the brain and retina), CRB2 (localized to the RPE, choroid, placenta, heart, lungs, and kidney), and CRB3 (expressed in a large variety of tissues).[114–116] Homozygous loss of CRB1 has been implicated in both LCA and RP, although the mechanism is unknown. A mouse model with a truncation of CRB1 displays shortened photoreceptor inner and outer segments, and the protein complex is believed to be involved in the maintenance of the cell's apico-basal polarity and adherens junctions.[117,118] Therefore, defects in structural proteins may lead to the malformation of the photoreceptor, as seen in *RDS* mutations, or cause changes in cell polarity and cell-cell interactions, as in the Crumbs mutations. However, the mechanism by which these mutations lead to photoreceptor degeneration remains unknown.

6.10. *Processing of messenger RNA and transcriptional defects*

Correct processing and transcription of messenger RNA (mRNA) are vital
to the development and function of photoreceptor cells. A genetic study of
Spanish families with adRP found six novel mutations in genes involved
in the splicing of introns during mRNA transcriptional processing.[119] This
process includes the spliceosome complex, composed of protein splicing
factors (PRPF3, PRPF8, and PRPF31), five small ribonuclear particles
(snRNPs), U1, U2, U4/6, and U5. U1 and U2 are responsible for recognition of splice sites, which are then cleaved by the tri-snRNP complex with
U4/6 and U5, which is recruited to the splice sites by the protein factors.[119,120] A mouse model with a *PRPF31* mutation displayed a loss of
RDS/peripherin expression, suggesting its role in RP disease.[120] However,
the mechanism by which these mRNA transcriptional components lead to
adRP is still unknown.

In Drosophila, an Otd homeodomain was determined to have an essential
role in photoreceptor development.[121] In mammalian systems, there are
three Otd-like homeodomains: OTX1, OTX2, and CRX. Each of these
mammalian homeodomains is known to regulate development of the posterior eye, and mutations in these genes are associated with LCA (*OTX2*
mutations) and RP (*CRX* mutations), as well as microphthalmia.[122,123] OTX2
and CRX appear to influence each other, as animal studies have shown that
Crx is a target of OTX2 and *Otx2* knockout mice also lack CRX expression.
Furthermore, CRX is known to regulate opsin molecules, and is associated
with cone-rod dystrophic diseases.[124] However, the function of CRX is not
yet determined, as it could either directly activate transcription or act
through other transcriptional regulators. It is believed that CRX may interact with protein complexes that modify histones, and therefore promote
chromatin remodeling in the cell.[120] It is necessary for further analysis to be
completed to understand the targets of these genes and how their regulation
of mRNA processing and transcription leads to photoreceptor dysfunction.

7. Summary

As witnessed in this chapter, the study of molecular genetics has greatly
assisted in the understanding of mechanisms of eye diseases. However,

much remains unknown about the exact manner in which gene mutations cause the loss of photoreceptor cells in retinal degenerative disease. Mammalian model systems and further characterization of gene functions *in vivo* will help to elucidate these mechanistic effects, as well as provide targets for drug and gene therapies to treat patients with eye diseases.

8. References

1. Gaillard, F. & Sauve, Y. Cell-based therapy for retinal degeneration: the promise of a cure. *Vis Res* **47**, 2815–2824 (2007).
2. J, G. Eye development. *Curr Top Dev Biol* **90**, 343–386 (2010).
3. Milhotra, A., Minja, F., Crum, A. & Burrowes, D. Ocular anatomy and cross-sectional imaging of the eye. *Semin Ultrasound CT MRI* **32**, 2–13 (2011).
4. Junquiera, L. & Carneiro, J. *Basic Histology: Text and Atlas*, 11 ed., McGraw-Hill, New York (2005).
5. Karan, G., Yang, Z., Howes, K., Zhao, Y., Chen, Y., Cameron, D.J., Lin, Y., Pearson, E. & Zhang, K. Loss of ER retention and sequestration of the wild-type ELOVL4 by Stargardt disease dominant negative mutants. *Mol Vis* **11**, 657–664 (2005).
6. D, B. The retinal pigment epithelium: a versatile partner in vision. *J Cell Sci Suppl* **17**, 189–195 (1993).
7. A, M. The polarity of the retinal pigment epithelium. *Traffic* **2**, 867–872 (2001).
8. L, R. Polarity and the development of the outer blood-retinal barrier. *Histol Histopathol* **12**, 1057–1067 (1997).
9. R, S. Interactions between the retinal pigment epithelium and the neural retina. *Doc Ophthalmol* **60**, 327–346 (1985).
10. K, P. Chemistry and biology of vision. *J Biol Chem* **287**, 1612–1619 (2012).
11. Tang, P., Kono, M., Koutalos, Y., Ablonczy, Z. & Crouch, R. New insights into retinoid metabolism and cycling within the retina. *Prog Retin Eye Res* **32**, 48–63 (2013).
12. Rivas, M. & Vecino, E. Animal models and different therapies for treatment of retinitis pigmentosa. *Histol Histopathol* **42**, 392–403 (2009).
13. Young, R. & Bok, D. Participation of the retinal pigment epithelium in the rod outer segment renewal process. *J Cell Biol* **42**, 392–403 (1969).
14. NG, B. Survival signaling in retinal pigment epithelial cells in response to oxidative stress: significance in retinal degenerations. *Adv Exp Med Biol* **572**, 531–540 (2006).

15. RH, C. Characteristics of photoreceptor PDE (PDE6): similarities and differences to PDE5. *Int J Impot Res* **16(suppl 1)**, S28–S33 (2004).
16. Fung, B., Hurley, J. & Stryer, L. Flow of information in the light-triggered cyclic nucleotide cascade of vision. *Proc Natl Acad Sci USA* **78**, 152–156 (1981).
17. Baehr, W., Devlin, M. & Applebury, M. Isolation and characterization of cGMP phosphodiesterase from bovine rod outer segments. *J Biol Chem* **254**, 11669–11677 (1979).
18. Colley, N.J., Baker, E.K., Stamnes, M.A. & Zuker, C.S. The cyclophilin homolog ninaA is required in the secretory pathway. *Cell* **67**, 255–263 (1991).
19. Deterre, P., Bigay, J., Forquet, F., Robert, M. & Chabre, M. cGMP phosphodiesterase of retinal rods is regulated by two inhibitory subunits. *Proc Natl Acad Sci USA* **85**, 2424–2428 (1988).
20. Miki, N., Baraban, J., Keirns, J., Boyce, J. & Bitensky, M. Purification and properties of the light-activated cyclic nucleotide phosphodiesterase of rod outer segments. *J Biol Chem* **250**, 6320–6327 (1975).
21. Palczewski, K., McDowell, J., Jakes, S., Ingebritsen, T. & Hargrave, P. Regulation of rhodopsin dephosphorylation by arrestin. *J Biol Chem* **264**, 15770–15773 (1989).
22. Arshavsky, V. & Bownds, M. Regulation of deactivation of photoreceptor G protein by its target enzyme and cGMP. *Nature* **357**, 416–417 (1992).
23. Bergsma, D. & Kaiser-Kupfer, M. A new form of albinism. *Am J Ophthalmol* **77**, 837–844 (1974).
24. Riess, O., Noerremoelle, A., Weber, B., Musarella, M.A. & Hayden, M.R. The search for mutations in the gene for the b subunit of the cGMP phosphodiesterase (PDEB) in patients with autosomal recessive retinitis pigmentosa. *Am J Hum Genet* **51**, 755–762 (1992).
25. Torre, V., Matthews, H. & Lamb, T. Role of calcium in regulating the cyclic GMP cascade of phototransduction in retinal rods. *Proc Natl Acad Sci USA* **83**, 7109–7113 (1986).
26. Lagnado, L. & Baylor, D. Signal flow in visual transduction. *Neuron* **8**, 995–1002 (1992).
27. KW, Y. Cyclic nucleotide-gated channels: an expanding new family of ion channels. *Proc Natl Acad Sci USA* **91**, 3481–3483 (1994).
28. K, P.G protein-coupled receptor rhodopsin. *Annu Rev Biochem* **75**, 743–767 (2006).
29. Yarfitz, S. & Hurley, J. Transduction mechanisms of vertebrate and invertebrate photoreceptors. *J Biol Chem* **269**, 14329–14332 (1994).

30. Blomhoff, R. & Blomhoff, H. Overview of retinoid metabolism and function. *J Neurobiol* **66**, 606–630 (2006).
31. van Soest, S., Westerveld, A., de Jong, P., Bleeker-Wagemakers, E. & Bergen, A. Retinitis pigmentosa: defined from a molecular point of view. *Surv Ophthalmol* **43**, 321–334 (1999).
32. Alstrom, C. & Olson, O. Heredo-retinopathia congenitalis monohybrida recessiva autosomalis. *Hereditas* **43**, 1–178 (1957).
33. Paunescu, K., Wabbels, B., Preising, M. & Lorenz, B. Longitudinal and cross sectional study of patients with early-onset severe retinal dystrophy associated with RPE65 mutations. *Graefes Arch Clin Exp Ophthalmol* **243**, 417–426 (2005).
34. Daiger, S., Rossiter, B., Greenberg, J., Christoffels, A. & Hide, W. Data services and software for identifying genes and mutations causing retinal degeneration. *Invest Ophthalmol Vis Sci* **39**, S295 (1998).
35. Dryja, T. & Berson, E. Retinitis pigmentosa and allied diseases: Implications of genetic heterogeneity. *Invest Opthalmol Vis Sci* **36**, 1197–1200 (1995).
36. Wang, D., Chan, W., Tam, P., Baum, L., Lam, D., Chong, K., Fan, B. & Pang, C. Gene mutations in retinitis pigmentosa and their clinical implications. *Clin Chim Acta* **351**, 5–16 (2005).
37. C, H. Retinitis pigmentosa. *Orphanet J Rare Dis* **1**, 40 (2006).
38. GE, H. Significance of abnormal pattern electroretinography in anterior visual pathway dysfunction. *Br J Ophthalmol* **71**, 166–171 (1987).
39. GE, H. Pattern electroretinography (PERG) and an integrated approach to visual pathway diagnosis. *Prog Retin Eye Res* **20**, 531–561 (2001).
40. Rodriguez de Turco, E.B., Deretic, D., Bazan, N.G. & Papermaster, D.S. Post-Golgi vesicles cotransport docosahexaenoyl-phospholipids and rhodopsin during frog photoreceptor membrane biogenesis. *J Biol Chem* **272**, 10491–10497 (1997).
41. Thompson, D., Gyurus, P., Fleischer, L., Bingham, E., McHenry, C., Apfelstedt-Sylla, E., Zrenner, E., Lorenz, B., Richards, J., Jacobson, S., Sieving, P. & Gal, A. Genetics and phenotypes of RPE65 mutations in inherited retinal degeneration. *Invest Ophthalmol Vis Sci* **41**, 4293–4299 (2000).
42. Morimura, H., Fishman, G., Grover, S., Fulton, A., Berson, E. & Dryja, T. Mutations in the RPE65 gene in patients with autosomal recessive retinitis pigmentosa or Leber congenital amaurosis. *Proc Natl Acad Sci USA* **95**, 3088–3093 (1998).
43. VA, M. *Mendelian Inheritance in Man*, The Johns Hopkins University Press, Baltimore (1994).

44. Pearson, P., Francomano, C., Foster, P., Bocchini, C., Li, P. & McKusick, V. The status of online Mendelian inheritance in man (OMIM) medio 1994. *Nucleic Acids Res* **22**, 3470–3473 (1994).

45. Hurley, J.B., Chertov, A., Lindsay, K., Giamarco, M., Cleghorn, W., Du, J. & Brockerhoff, S. Energy Metabolism in the Vertebrate Retina. In *Vertebrate Photoreceptors* (Furukawa, T., Hurley, J. B. & Kawamura, S. eds.), Springer Japan. pp. 91–137 (2014).

46. Linsenmeier, R.A. Effects of light and darkness on oxygen distribution and consumption in the cat retina. *J Gen Physiol* **88**, 521–542 (1986).

47. Ahmed, J., Braun, R.D., Dunn, R. & Linsenmeier, R.A. Oxygen distribution in the macaque retina. *Invest Ophthalmol Vis Sci* **34**, 516–521 (1993).

48. Birol, G., Wang, S., Budzynski, E., Wangsa-Wirawan, N. D. & Linsenmeier, R.A. Oxygen distribution and consumption in the macaque retina. *Am J Physiol Heart Circ Physiol* **293**, H1696–1704 (2007).

49. Yau, K.W. Phototransduction mechanism in retinal rods and cones. The Friedenwald Lecture. *Invest Ophthalmol Vis Sci* **35**, 9–32 (1994).

50. Wong-Riley, M.T. Energy metabolism of the visual system. *Eye Brain* **2**, 99–116 (2010).

51. Feigl, B. Age-related maculopathy — linking aetiology and pathophysiological changes to the ischaemia hypothesis. *Prog Retin Eye Res* **28**, 63–86 (2009).

52. Owsley, C., Jackson, G.R., Cideciyan, A.V., Huang, Y., Fine, S.L., Ho, A.C., Maguire, M.G., Lolley, V. & Jacobson, S. G. Psychophysical evidence for rod vulnerability in age-related macular degeneration. *Invest Ophthalmol Vis Sci* **41**, 267–273 (2000).

53. Marín-Hernández, A., Gallardo-Pérez, J.C., Ralph, S.J., Rodríguez-Enríquez, S. & Moreno-Sánchez, R. HIF-1alpha modulates energy metabolism in cancer cells by inducing over-expression of specific glycolytic isoforms. *Mini Rev Med Chem* **9**, 1084–1101 (2009).

54. Kim, J.W., Tchernyshyov, I., Semenza, G.L. & Dang, C.V. HIF-1-mediated expression of pyruvate dehydrogenase kinase: a metabolic switch required for cellular adaptation to hypoxia. *Cell Metab* **3**, 177–185 (2006).

55. Semenza, G.L. Targeting HIF-1 for cancer therapy. *Nat Rev Cancer* **3**, 721–732 (2003).

56. Semenza, G.L. HIF-1: upstream and downstream of cancer metabolism. *Curr Opin Genet Dev* **20**, 51–56 (2010).

57. Zhang, H., He, S., Spee, C., Ishikawa, K. & Hinton, D.R. SIRT1 mediated inhibition of VEGF/VEGFR2 signaling by Resveratrol and its relevance to choroidal neovascularization. *Cytokine* (2015).

58. Sweigard, J.H., Matsumoto, H., Smith, K.E., Kim, L.A., Paschalis, E.I., Okonuki, Y., Castillejos, A., Kataoka, K., Hasegawa, E., Yanai, R., Husain, D., Lambris, J.D., Vavvas, D., Miller, J.W. & Connor, K.M. Inhibition of the alternative complement pathway preserves photoreceptors after retinal injury. *Sci Transl Med* **7**, 297ra116 (2015).

59. Ding, J.-D., Kelly, U., Groelle, M., Christenbury, J.G., Zhang, W. & Rickman, C.B. The Role of Complement Dysregulation in AMD Mouse Models. in *Retinal Degenerative Diseases* (Ash, J., Grimm, C., Hollyfield, J.G., & Anderson, R.E., LaVail, M.M. & Rickman, C.B. eds.), Springer, New York. pp. 213–219 (2014).

60. Toomey, C.B., Kelly, U., Saban, D.R. & Bowes Rickman, C. Regulation of age-related macular degeneration-like pathology by complement factor H. *Proc Natl Acad Sci USA* **112**, E3040–3049 (2015).

61. Boon, C., Jeroen Klevering, B., Keunen, J., Hoyng, C. & Theelen, T. Fundus autofluorescence imaging of retinal dystrophies. *Vis Res* **48**, 2569–2577 (2008).

62. Sparrow, J. & Boulton, M. RPE lipofuscin and its role in retinal pathobiology. *Exp Eye Res* **80**, 595–606 (2005).

63. Zhou, J., Jang, Y., Kim, S. & Sparrow, J. Complement activation by photooxidation products of A2E, a lipofuscin constituent of the retinal pigment epithelium. *Proc Natl Acad Sci USA* **103**, 16182–16187 (2006).

64. Sparrow, J., Cai, B., Jang, Y., Zhou, J. & Nakanishi, K. A2E, a fluorophore of RPE lipofuscin, can destabilize membrane. *Adv Exp Med Biol* **572**, 63–68 (2006).

65. Lakkaraju, A., Finnemann, S. & Rodriguez-Boulan, E. The lipofuscin fluorophore A2E perturbs cholesterol metabolism in retinal pigment epithelial cells. *Proc Natl Acad Sci USA* **104**, 11026–11031 (2007).

66. Sparrow, J. & Cai, B. Blue light-induced apoptosis of A2E-containing RPE: involvement of caspase-3 and protection by Bcl-2. *Invest Ophthalmol Vis Sci* **42**, 1356–1362 (2001).

67. Sparrow, J., Fishkin, N., Zhou, J., Cai, B., Jang, Y., Krane, S., Itagaki, Y. & Nakanishi, K. A2E, a by product of the visual cycle. *Vis Res* **43**, 2983–2990 (2003).

68. Weiter, J., Delori, F., Wing, G. & Fitch, K. Retinal pigment epithelial lipofuscin and melanin and choroidal melanin in human eyes. *Invest Ophthalmol Vis Sci* **27**, 145–152 (1986).

69. Fain, G. & Lisman, J. Photoreceptor degeneration in vitamin A deprivation and retinitis pigmentosa: the equivalent light hypothesis. *Exp Eye Res* **57**, 335–340 (1993).

70. Burns, M. & Baylor, D. Activation, deactivation, and adaptation in vertebrate photoreceptor cells. *Annu Rev Neurosci* **24**, 779–805 (2001).

71. Reed, J., Talwar, H., Cuddy, M., Baffy, G., Williamson, J., Rapp, U. & Fisher, G. Mitochondrial protein p26 BCL2 reduces growth factor requirements of NIH3T3 fibroblasts. *Exp Cell Res* **195**, 277–283 (1991).

72. Woodruff, M., Wang, Z., Chung, H., Redmond, T., Fain, G. & Lem, J. Spontaneous activity of opsin apoprotein is a cause of Leber congenital amaurosis. *Nat Genet* **35**, 158–164 (2003).

73. Lisman, J. & Fain, G. Support for the equivalent light hypothesis for RP. *Nat Med* **1**, 1254–1255 (1995).

74. Fain, G. & Lisman, J. Light, Ca2+, and photoreceptor death: new evidence for the equivalent-light hypothesis from arrestin knockout mice. *Invest Ophthalmol Vis Sci* **40**, 2770–2772 (1999).

75. Wang, H., Pathan, N., Ethell, I., Krajewski, S., Yamaguchi, Y., Shibasaki, F., McKeon, F., Bobo, T., Franke, T. & Reed, J. Ca^{2+}-induced apoptosis through calcineurin dephosphorylation of BAD. *Science* **284**, 339–343 (1999).

76. Lin, J. H., Walter, P. & Yen, T. S. Endoplasmic reticulum stress in disease pathogenesis. *Annu Rev Pathol* **3**, 399–425 (2008).

77. Tabas, I. & Ron, D. Integrating the mechanisms of apoptosis induced by endoplasmic reticulum stress. *Nat Cell Biol* **13**, 184–190 (2011).

78. Lin, J.H. & Lavail, M.M. Misfolded proteins and retinal dystrophies. *Adv Exp Med Biol* **664**, 115–121 (2010).

79. Berson, E.L., Rosner, B., Sandberg, M.A., Hayes, K.C., Nicholson, B.W., Weigel-DiFrano, C. & Willett, W. Vitamin A supplementation for retinitis pigmentosa. *Archives of ophthalmology* **111**, 1456–1459 (1993).

80. Chiang, W.C., Hiramatsu, N., Messah, C., Kroeger, H. & Lin, J.H. Selective activation of ATF6 and PERK endoplasmic reticulum stress signaling pathways prevent mutant rhodopsin accumulation. *Invest Ophthalmol Vis Sci* **53**, 7159–7166 (2012).

81. Gorbatyuk, M.S., Knox, T., LaVail, M.M., Gorbatyuk, O.S., Noorwez, S.M., Hauswirth, W.W., Lin, J.H., Muzyczka, N. & Lewin, A.S. Restoration of visual function in P23H rhodopsin transgenic rats by gene delivery of BiP/Grp78. *Proc Natl Acad Sci USA* **107**, 5961–5966 (2010).

82. Kunte, M.M., Choudhury, S., Manheim, J.F., Shinde, V.M., Miura, M., Chiodo, V.A., Hauswirth, W.W., Gorbatyuk, O.S. & Gorbatyuk, M.S. ER stress is involved in T17M rhodopsin-induced retinal degeneration. *Invest Ophthalmol Vis Sci* **53**, 3792–3800 (2012).

83. Lin, J.H., Li, H., Yasumura, D., Cohen, H.R., Zhang, C., Panning, B., Shokat, K.M., Lavail, M.M. & Walter, P. IRE1 signaling affects cell fate during the unfolded protein response. *Science* **318**, 944–949 (2007).
84. Shinde, V.M., Sizova, O.S., Lin, J.H., Lavail, M.M. & Gorbatyuk, M.S. ER Stress in Retinal Degeneration in S334ter Rho Rats. *PLoS One* **7**, e33266 (2012).
85. Tam, B.M. & Moritz, O.L. Characterization of rhodopsin P23H-induced retinal degeneration in a Xenopus laevis model of retinitis pigmentosa. *Invest Ophthalmol Vis Sci* **47**, 3234–3241 (2006).
86. Kroeger, H., Messah, C., Ahern, K., Gee, J., Joseph, V., Matthes, M.T., Yasumura, D., Gorbatyuk, M.S., Chiang, W.C., LaVail, M.M. & Lin, J.H. Induction of endoplasmic reticulum stress genes, BiP and chop, in genetic and environmental models of retinal degeneration. *Invest Ophthalmol Vis Sci* **53**, 7590–7599 (2012).
87. Yang, L.P., Wu, L.M., Guo, X.J., Li, Y. & Tso, M.O. Endoplasmic reticulum stress is activated in light-induced retinal degeneration. *J Neurosci Res* **86**, 910–919 (2008).
88. Yang, L.P., Wu, L.M., Guo, X.J. & Tso, M.O. Activation of endoplasmic reticulum stress in degenerating photoreceptors of the rd1 mouse. *Invest Ophthalmol Vis Sci* **48**, 5191–5198 (2007).
89. Wang, T. & Chen, J. Induction of the Unfolded Protein Response by Constitutive G-protein Signaling in Rod Photoreceptor Cells. *J Biological Chem* **289**, 29310–29321 (2014).
90. Kohl, S., Zobor, D., Chiang, W.C., Weisschuh, N., Staller, J., Menendez, I.G., Chang, S., Beck, S.C., Garcia Garrido, M., Sothilingam, V., Seeliger, M.W., Stanzial, F., Benedicenti, F., Inzana, F., Héon, E., Vincent, A., Beis, J., Strom, T.M., Rudolph, G., Roosing, S., Hollander, A.I., Cremers, F.P., Lopez, I., Ren, H., Moore, A.T., Webster, A.R., Michaelides, M., Koenekoop, R.K., Zrenner, E., Kaufman, R.J., Tsang, S.H., Wissinger, B. & Lin, J.H. Mutations in the unfolded protein response regulator ATF6 cause the cone dysfunction disorder achromatopsia. *Nat Genet* **47**, 757–765 (2015).
91. Hiramatsu, N., Messah, C., Han, J., Lavail, M. M., Kaufman, R. J. & Lin, J.H. Translational and Post-Translational Regulation of XIAP by eIF2alpha and ATF4 promotes ER stress-induced Cell Death during the Unfolded Protein Response. *Mol Biol Cell* (2014).
92. Ryoo, H.D., Domingos, P.M., Kang, M.J. & Steller, H. Unfolded protein response in a Drosophila model for retinal degeneration. *EMBO J* **26**, 242–252 (2007).

93. Yang, P., Peairs, J.J., Tano, R., Zhang, N., Tyrell, J. & Jaffe, G.J. Caspase-8-mediated apoptosis in human RPE cells. *Invest Ophthalmol Vis Sci* **48**, 3341–3349 (2007).
94. Chiang, W.C., Kroeger, H., Sakami, S., Messah, C., Yasumura, D., Matthes, M.T., Coppinger, J.A., Palczewski, K., LaVail, M.M. & Lin, J.H. Robust Endoplasmic Reticulum-Associated Degradation of Rhodopsin Precedes Retinal Degeneration. *Mol Neurobiol* (2014).
95. Chiang, W.C., Messah, C. & Lin, J.H. IRE1 directs proteasomal and lysosomal degradation of misfolded rhodopsin. *Mol Biol Cell* **23**, 758–770 (2012).
96. Lobanova, E.S., Finkelstein, S., Skiba, N.P. & Arshavsky, V.Y. Proteasome overload is a common stress factor in multiple forms of inherited retinal degeneration. *Proc Natl Acad Sci USA* 110, 9986–9991 (2013).
97. Adams, N., Awadein, A. & Toma, H. The retinal ciliopathies. *Ophthalmic Genet* **28**, 113–125 (2007).
98. PL, B. Lifting the lid on Pandora's box: the Bardet-Biedl syndrome. *Curr Opin Genet Dev* 15, 315–323 (2005).
99. Blacque, O. & Leroux, M. Bardet-Biedl syndrome: an emerging pathomechanism of intracellular transport. *Cell Mol Life Sci* 63, 2145–2161 (2006).
100. Nishimura, D., Fath, M., Mullins, R., Searby, C. &rews, M., Davis, R. Andorf, J., Mykytyn, K., Swiderski, R., Yang, B., Carmi, R., Stone, E. & Sheffield, V. Bbs2-null mice have neurosensory deficits, a defect in social dominance, and retinopathy associated with mislocalization of rhodopsin. *Proc Natl Acad Sci USA* **101**, 16588–16593 (2004).
101. Mockel, A., Obringer, C., Hakvoort, T.B., Seeliger, M., Lamers, W.H., Stoetzel, C., Dollfus, H. & Marion, V. Pharmacological modulation of the retinal unfolded protein response in Bardet-Biedl syndrome reduces apoptosis and preserves light detection ability. *J Biol Chem* **287**, 37483–37494 (2012).
102. Sharon, D., Sandberg, M., Rabe, V., Stillberger, M., Dryja, T. & Berson, E. RP2 and RPGR mutations and clinical correlations in patients with X-linked retinitis pigmentosa. *Am J Hum Genet* 73, 1131–1146 (2003).
103. Shu, X., McDowall, E., Brown, A. & Wright, A. The human retinitis pigmentosa GTPase regulator gene variant database. *Hum Mutat* 29, 605–608 (2008).
104. PA, F. Insights into X-linked retinitis pigmentosa type 3, allied diseases and underlying pathomechanisms. *Hum Mol Genet* **14 Spec No. 2**, R259–267 (2005).

105. Neidhardt, J., Glaus, E., Barthelmes, D., Zeitz, C., Fleischhauer, J. & Berger, W. Identification and characterization of a novel RPGR isoform in human retina. *Hum Mutat* **28**, 797–807 (2007).
106. Vervoort, R. & Wright, A. Mutations of RPGR in X-linked retinitis pigmentosa (RP3). *Hum Mutat* **19**, 486–500 (2002).
107. Alexandrov, K., Horiuchi, H., Steele-Mortimer, O., Seabra, M. & Zerial, M. Rab escort protein-1 is a multifunctional protein that accompanies newly prenylated rab proteins to their target membranes. *EMBO J* **13**, 5262–5273 (1994).
108. Krock, B., Bilotta, J. & Perkins, B. Noncell-autonomous photoreceptor degeneration in a zebrafish model of choroideremia. *Proc Natl Acad Sci USA* **104**, 4600–4605 (2007).
109. RK, K. Choroideremia is caused by a defective phagocytosis by the RPE of photoreceptor disc membranes, not by an intrinsic photoreceptor defect. *Ophthalmic Genet* **28**, 185–186 (2007).
110. Leroy, B., Kailasanathan, A., De Laey, J., Black, G. & Manson, F. Intrafamilial phenotypic variability in families with RDS mutations: exclusion of ROM1 as a genetic modifier for those with retinitis pigmentosa. *Br J Ophthalmol* **91**, 89–93 (2007).
111. Dalke, C. & Graw, J. Mouse mutants as models for congenital retinal disorders. *Exp Eye Res* **81**, 503–512 (2005).
112. Sanyal, S. & Jansen, H. Absence of receptor outer segments in the retina of rds mutant mice. *Neurosci Lett* **21**, 23–26 (1981).
113. Dejneka, N., Rex, T. & Bennett, J. Gene therapy and animal models for retinal disease. *Dev Ophthalmol* **37**, 188–198 (2003).
114. Makarova, O., Roh, M., Liu, C., Laurinec, S. & Margolis, B. Mammalian Crumbs3 is a small transmembrane protein linked to protein associated with Lin-7 (Pals1). *Gene* **302**, 21–29 (2003).
115. van den Hurk, J., Rashbass, P., Roepman, R., Davis, J., Voesenek, K., Arends, M., Zonneveld, M., van Roekel, M., Cameron, K., Rohrschneider, K., Heckenlively, J., Koenekoop, R., Hoyng, C., Cremers, F. & den Hollander, A. Characterization of the Crumbs homolog 2 (CRB2) gene and analysis of its role in retinitis pigmentosa and Leber congenital amaurosis. *Mol Vis* **11**, 263–273 (2005).
116. den Hollander, A., Ghiani, M., de Kok, Y., Wijnholds, J., Ballabio, A., Cremers, F. & Broccoli, V. Isolation of Crb1, a mouse homologue of Drosophila crumbs, and analysis of its expression pattern in eye and brain. *Mech Dev* **110**, 203–207 (2002).

117. Gosens, I., den Hollander, A., Cremers, F. & Roepman, R. Composition and function of the Crumbs protein complex in the mammalian retina. *Exp Eye Res* **86**, 713–726 (2008).

118. Mehalow, A., Kameya, S., Smith, R., Hawes, N., Denegre, J., Young, J., Bechtold, L., Haider, N., Tepass, U., Heckenlively, J., Chang, B., Naggert, J. & Nishina, P. CRB1 is essential for external limiting membrane integrity and photoreceptor morphogenesis in the mammalian retina. *Hum Mol Genet* **12**, 2179–2189 (2003).

119. Martinez-Gimeno, M., Gamundi, M., Hernan, I., Maseras, M., Milla, E., Ayuso, C., Garcia-Sandoval, B., Beneyto, M., Vilela, C., Baiget, M., Antinolo, G. & Carballo, M. Mutations in the pre-mRNA splicing-factor genes PRPF3, PRPF8, and PRPF31 in Spanish families with autosomal dominant retinitis pigmentosa. *Invest Ophthalmol Vis Sci* **44**, 2171–2177 (2003).

120. Mordes, D., Yuan, L., Xu, L., Kawada, M., Molday, R. & Wu, J. Identification of photoreceptor genes affected by PRPF31 mutations associated with autosomal dominant retinitis pigmentosa. *Neurobiol Dis* **26**, 291–300 (2007).

121. Plouhinec, J., Sauka-Spengler, T., Germot, A., Le Mentec, C., Cabana, T., Harrison, G., Pieau, C., Sire, J., Veron, G. & Mazan, S. The mammalian Crx genes are highly divergent representatives of the Otx5 gene family, a gnathostome orthology class of orthodenticle-related homeogenes involved in the differentiation of retinal photoreceptors and circadian entrainment. *Mol Biol Evol* **20**, 513–521 (2003).

122. Hennig, A., Peng, G. & Chen, S. Regulation of photoreceptor gene expression by Crx-associated transcription factor network. *Brain Res* **1192**, 114–133 (2008).

123. Nolen, L., Amor, D., Haywood, A., St Heaps, L., Willcock, C., Mehelec, M., Tam, P., Billson, F., Grigg, J., Peters, G. & Jamieson, R. Deletion at 14q22–23 indicates a contiguous gene syndrome comprising anophthalmia, pituitary hypoplasia, and ear anomalies. *Am J Med Genet A* **140**, 1711–1718 (2006).

124. Kitiratschky, V., Nagy, D., Zabel, T., Zrenner, E., Wissinger, B., Kohl, S. & Jagle, H. Cone and cone-rod dystrophy segregating in the same pedigree due to the same novel CRX gene mutation. *Br J Ophthalmol* **92**, 1086–1091 (2008).

Chapter 2: Ophthalmic Imaging

Colin S. Tan[*,†] *and Srinivas R. Sadda*[‡]

* *National Healthcare Group Eye Institute,*
Tan Tock Seng Hospital, Singapore

[†] *Fundus Image Reading Center,*
National Healthcare Group Eye Institute, Singapore

[‡] *Doheny Eye Institute, University of California Los Angeles, USA*

1. Introduction

Ophthalmic imaging plays an essential role in the diagnosis, monitoring and treatment of various ocular diseases, especially those involving the posterior pole. The continuous development of new modalities, as well as rapid advances in existing modalities, have led to significant expansion of the scope of ophthalmic imaging and considerable improvements in the ability of ophthalmologists to image the retina. Many of these imaging modalities are complementary and provide a broad array of diagnostic information to the clinician.

In this chapter, we will explore the common imaging modalities available to ophthalmologists, explain the basic imaging principles, and also illustrate the interpretation of these imaging techniques in common ocular diseases.

Financial disclosures:

Colin S. Tan — Research Support from National Healthcare Group Clinician Scientist Career Scheme Grant CSCS 12/005. Conference support from Bayer, Heidelberg Engineering, Novartis.

SriniVas R. Sadda — Consultant for Allegan, Genentech, Roche, Regeneron, Alcon, Bausch & Lomb, Optos and Carl Zeiss Meditec. Research Support from Allegan, Genentech, Optos, and Carl Zeiss Meditec.

2. Fluorescein Angiography

2.1. *Principles of fluorescein angiography*

Fluorescein angiography (FA) is an imaging technique used to visualize vascular abnormalities within the retinal circulation. The basis of FA (and indocyanine green angiography, discussed later) is the principle of fluorescence, which occurs when a chemical absorbs electromagnetic energy of a certain wavelength and re-emits this at a longer wavelength of lower energy levels.

Fluorescein has an absorption spectrum between 465 nm to 490 nm, which lies within the blue end of the spectrum, while its emission spectrum lies between 520 nm to 530 nm, in the green range. When injected intravenously, between 70 to 80% of the dye is bound by plasma proteins, whereas the remaining unbound portion is free to diffuse through vessel walls. Since structures such as normal retinal vessels and the retinal pigment epithelium normally prevent diffusion of fluorescein molecules, FA is an ideal modality to image the retinal circulation. Unbound fluorescein, however, leaks readily through the fenestrations of the choriocapillaris, which renders FA unsuitable for imaging of the choroidal circulation.

FA can be performed using modified fundus cameras or confocal scanning laser ophthalmoscopes (CSLO). Using modified fundus cameras, a bright light source is used to illuminate the entire fundus simultaneously and the sum total of the reflected light is captured by the photographic film or, more commonly in the current era, a charge-coupled device (CCD) camera. Appropriate barrier filters are used to modify the wavelengths of the illuminating light, while allowing absorption of light only within the emission spectrum.

Using CSLO, light from a laser source is scanned successively in a horizontal direction, then displaced vertically with a tilting mirror, performing the imaging using a series of rapid horizontal sweeps in a raster fashion. A small pinhole ensures that only light from a specific focal plane (for example, the retina) is allowed to pass through to the detector, thereby allowing precise delineation of a thin layer of the retina without interference from reflected light from structures that are either deeper or more superficial. This is in contrast to modified fundus cameras, where the various vascular layers are superimposed on top of one another.

2.2. Interpretation of fluorescein angiography

In order to better understand abnormalities in fluorescein angiography, it is essential to be familiar with the appearance of a normal fluorescein angiogram. After injection of fluorescein, the dye first appears within the large choroidal vessels and choriocapillaris. Due to leakage from the fenestrations of the choriocapillaris, there is diffuse background fluorescence, preventing visualization of the individual choroidal vessels. Shortly thereafter, the fluorescein dye appears within the retinal circulation, then fills up the venous circulation — initially in a lamellar pattern (lamellar flow).

Abnormalities in fluorescein angiography consist of either hyperfluorescence (increased levels of fluorescence) and hypofluorescence (decreased levels of fluorescence). The common causes of each are listed below:

Hyperfluorescence:

* Leakage
* Pooling
* Staining of scars and other tissues
* Retinal pigment epithelium window defect
* Neovascularization (Abnormal new vessels)

Hyperfluorescence refers to an increased level of fluorescence relative to the expected normal fluorescence for that region at that point in the angiogram. **Leakage** occurs from abnormal blood vessels either within the retina or choroid, and is characterized by increase in both size and intensity of the hyperfluorescence over time (Figs. 1 and 2). In some cases, abnormal vessels, especially more chronic/older lesions, may not demonstrate significant leakage. In these cases, the **abnormal new vessels** themselves (e.g. retinal angiomatous proliferation) are sources of hyperfluorescence. Pooling occurs when the fluorescein dye accumulates over time within an enclosed anatomical space, such as underneath a serous retinal detachment (Fig. 3) or an elevation of the retinal pigment epithelium (pigment epithelial detachment). **Staining** refers to an accumulation of dye within tissue, such as scar tissue. In both pooling and staining, the intensity of the hyperfluorescence increases over time, but not the size, since the fluorescein dye accumulates within a localized

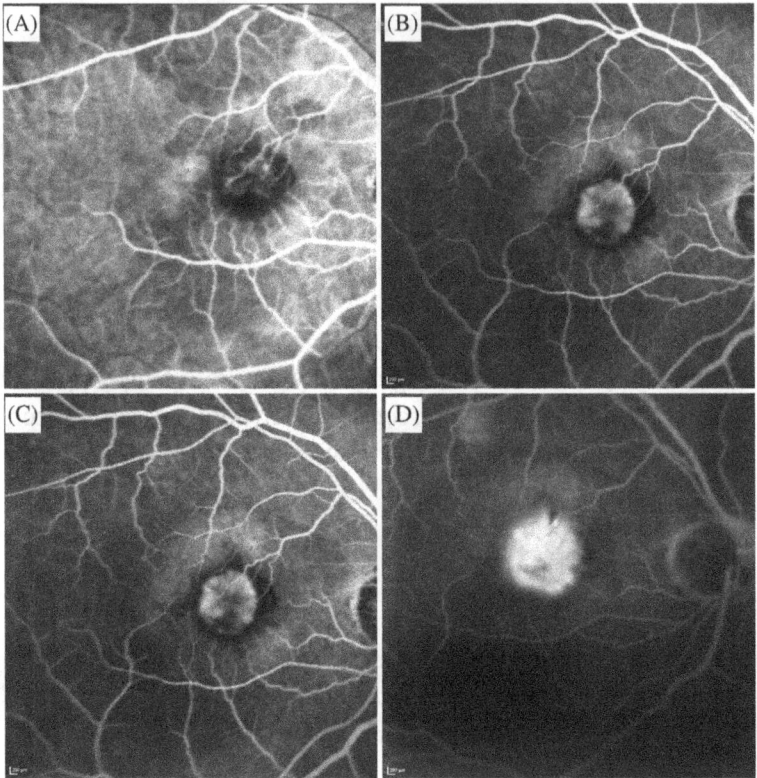

Figure 1. Fluorescein angiogram (FA) demonstrating leakage from classic choroidal neovascularization (CNV). (A) Early phase angiogram at 14 s demonstrating filling of abnormal vessels in a lacy pattern. (B) Angiogram at 45 s showing complete filling of the CNV. (C) FA at 5 min showing increased intensity of the area of hyperfluorescence. (D) Late phase angiogram at 10 min. Both the size and intensity of the hyperfluorescent area have increased relative to the early phases, and the borders of the lesion are indistinct.

region. A **window defect** in the retinal pigment epithelium (due to atrophy, for example) would result in increased transmission of the fluorescence, resulting in hyperfluorescence. This region is usually sharply defined and corresponds with the boundaries of the atrophy seen on colour fundus photography. The hyperfluorescence does not increase in size throughout the angiogram and its intensity may fluctuate over the course of the angiogram due to recirculation of the dye.

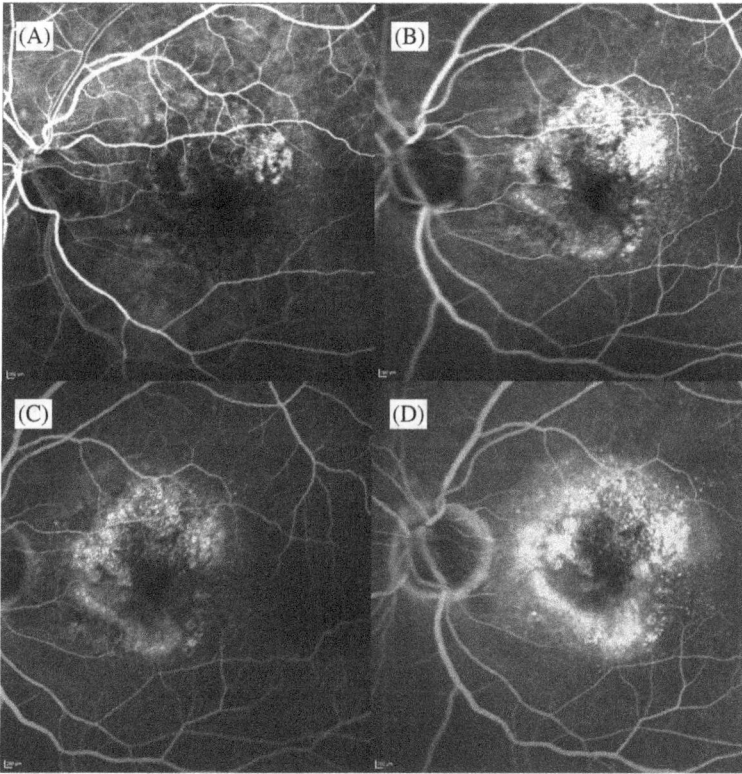

Figure 2. Fluorescein angiogram (FA) demonstrating leakage from occult choroidal neovascularization. (A) Early phase FA at 17 s demonstrating areas of increased fluorescence superior to the fovea. The source of the leakage is less distinct compared to classic CNV. (B) FA at 1 min. Both the area and intensity of hyperfluorescence have increased. (C) FA at 4 min. (D) FA at 20 min showing further increases in both area and intensity of hyperfluorescence, especially inferiorly.

Hypofluorescence:

- Vascular filling defects
- Blocked fluorescence

Hypofluorescence refers to decreased amounts of fluorescence relative to normal. Areas of reduced or absent perfusion are characterized by

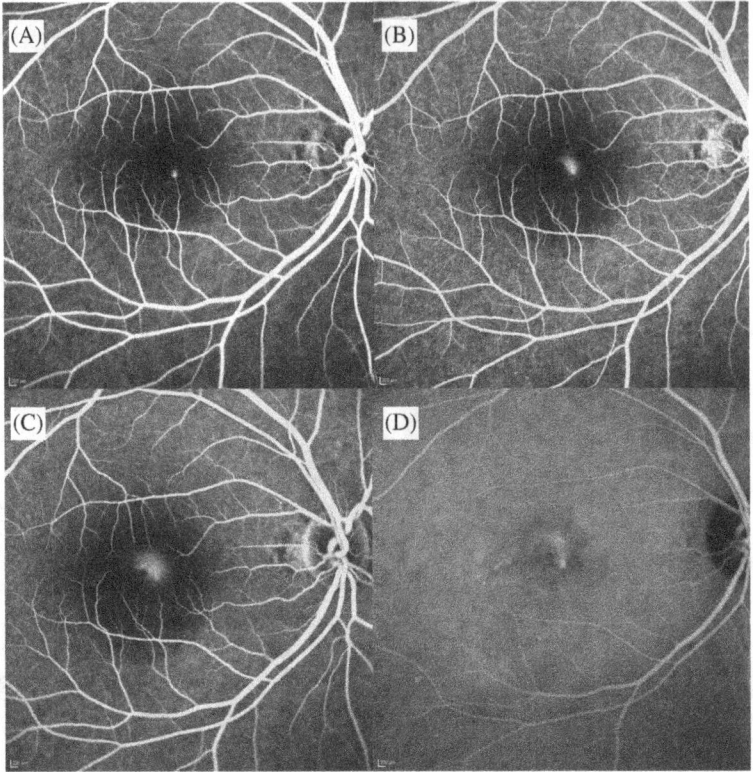

Figure 3.   Central serous chorioretinopathy. (A) Fluorescein angiogram at 42 s, demonstrating pinpoint hyperfluorescence. (B) FA at 3 min. The hypefluorescence has increased and spread superiorly. (C) FA at 10 min, demonstrating pooling of the dye within the subretinal space, typically described as a "smokestack" appearance. (D) Indocyanine green angiogram taken at 5 min. Areas of increased fluorescence correspond to the area of leakage seen on FA. There are additional areas of hyperfluorescence temporal to the fovea, which are believed to represent defects in the retinal pigment epithelium. The underlying choroidal vessels are indistinct, due to choroidal vascular hyperpermeability.

a **vascular filling defect** which have clear and distinct boundaries, corresponding to the area of non-perfusion (Fig. 4). These tend to coincide with anatomical boundaries of the blood vessels and their supplied territories. Transmission of the dye may be reduced or obstructed (i.e. "**blocked**") by the presence of abnormal blocking material, such as preretinal, intraretinal, subretinal blood or a very dense scar. These

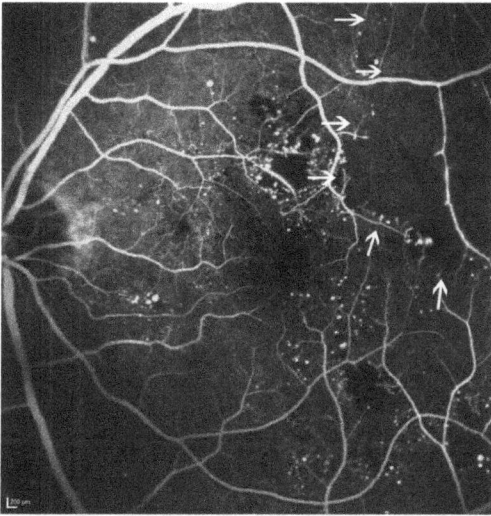

Figure 4. Fluorescein angiogram of a patient with diabetic retinopathy. A large area of capillary dropout is indicated by white arrows. Other small areas of capillary dropout are seen superior and infero-temporal to the fovea. Multiple points of hyperfluorescence from microaneurysms are seen throughout the fundus.

result in reduced fluorescence that correspond to the blocking abnormality and do not respect vascular landmarks or distributions (Fig. 5).

2.2.1. Age-related macular degeneration (AMD)

Fluorescein angiography is a critical tool in the diagnosis of neovascular AMD and was used extensively in the early landmark studies such as the Macular Photocoagulation study[1] and the Treatment of AMD with Photodynamic Therapy (TAP)[2] and Verteporfin in Photodynamic Therapy (VIP)[3,4] studies. Initially, the angiograms were performed using flash photographic systems, although CSLO systems are now commonly used in many centers. These early studies defined specific angiographic sub-types of CNV lesions based on their appearance.[1,4,5]

Classic CNV is defined by the presence of bright, well-demarcated, fairly homogenous areas of hyperfluorescence which appear in the early phases

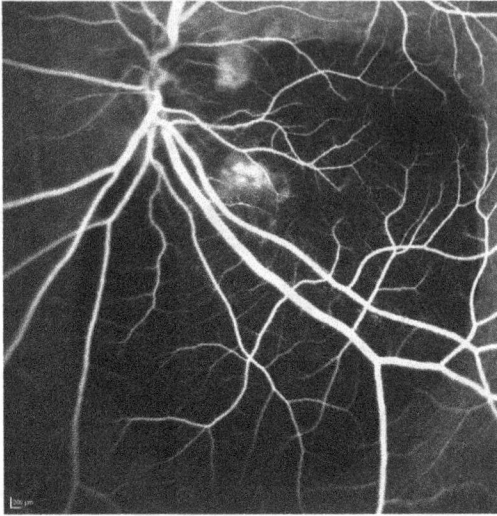

Figure 5. Fluorescein angiogram demonstrating blocked fluorescence (an area of reduced fluorescence compared to what is normal for that region) extending from the optic disc to the fovea and inferiorly. An area of hyperfluorescence is seen within this region, just superior to the infero-temporal arcades. This represents leakage from choroidal neovascularization.

of the angiogram (Fig. 1). Sometimes in the very early phases, fine choroidal new vessels can be seen, which is often described as a "lacy" or "cartwheel" appearance, although identification of the actual new vessels is not required to make a diagnosis of classic CNV. Subsequently, in the mid and late phases of the angiogram, there is progressive increase in both the size and intensity of the hyperfluorescence due to leakage. This obscures the precise boundaries of the original CNV lesion. OCT correlation studies have revealed that classic CNV is typically located in the sub-neurosensory retinal space, and thus consistent with histologic Type 1 CNV.

Occult CNV is believed to lie beneath the retinal pigment epithelium and hence is more difficult to distinguish from the surrounding choroiocapillaries, with no clearly identifiable vessels (Fig. 2). Occult CNV occurs in two forms. One form is that of a fibrovascular pigment epithelium detachment (fvPED). This consists of an area of stippled hyperfluorescence, often with a granular appearance, appearing within the first 1 to 2 minutes of the angiogram. The region is irregularly elevated, a feature best appreciated on stereoscopic examination. In later phases, the hyperfluorescence increases due to pooling of the dye underneath the RPE, however this is often not as intense as in classic CNV. In addition, there could be leakage surrounding the fvPED due to the presence of subretinal fluid. The other form of occult CNV is termed late leakage of undetermined source (LLUS). The leakage typically appears in the late phases of the angiogram (2 to 5 minutes) and is characterized by speckled areas of leakage with indistinct boundaries and no apparent source seen during the early phases. Recently it was demonstrated by OCT correlation that the difference in these two forms of Occult CNV is due to the level of elevation of the overlying RPE, with areas of LLUS representing a shallower elevation.[6] These OCT correlation studies have also revealed that occult CNV is invariably located in the sub-RPE space, and thus consistent with histologic Type 1 CNV.

3. Indocyanine Green Angiography

3.1. *Principles of indocyanine green angiography*

Indocyanine green functions very much like fluorescein angiography, but is commonly used to image the choroidal circulation, including choroidal neovascular membranes, in diseases such as AMD and polypoidal choroidal vasculopathy (Fig. 6). The principles underlying indocyanine green angiography (ICGA) share many similarities with fluorescein angiography, and ICGA can be performed using either flash fundus photography or confocal scanning laser ophthalmoscopy.

One of the key differences in ICGA is the dye. The absorption (790 nm to 805 nm) and emission (825 nm to 835 nm) both lie in the infrared spectrum.[7] This allows greater penetration through tissues that contain pigment, such as the retinal pigment epithelium or hemorrhages. Where there is blockage of the light in fluorescein angiography, the use of indocyanine green allows greater visualization of the structures beneath the obstruction.

Another useful feature of indocyanine green is that it has a higher affinity for plasma proteins — up to 98% of indocyanine green is protein

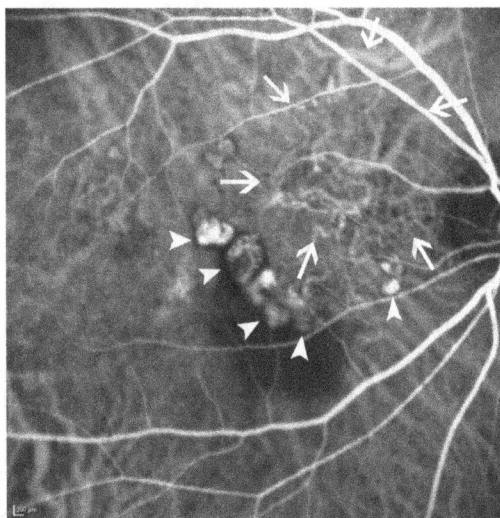

Figure 6. Polypoidal choroidal vasculopathy. The indocyanine-green angiogram shows large polyps (arrowheads) supplied by a branching vascular network (outlined by arrows).

bound. Consequently, this dye does not leak from the choriocapillaris, thus allowing clear visualization of the choroidal circulation.[7]

3.2. Interpretation of indocyanine green angiography

During ICGA, both the large choroidal vessels and retinal vessels are clearly seen during the early phases. Subsequently, these become less distinct during the late phase of the angiograms. Throughout the various phases of the angiogram, the optic disc is dark which is in contrast to fluorescein angiography.

Increases in fluorescence during angiography are usually due to abnormal vasculature, such as the choroidal neovascular membrane in AMD, or the polyps and branching vascular networks in polypoidal choroidal vasculopathy.

Earlier studies have used certain terms to describe findings on indocyanine green angiography:[8]

- **Focal spots (hot spots):** These are bright, hyperfluorescent lesions less than one disc area in size.

- **Plaques**: These are large areas of hyperfluorescence (greater than one disc area in size), which usually occur subfoveally, and correspond to the CNV lesion.
- **Combined lesions**: Some lesions manifest with both focal spots and plaques, which can either be confluent or distinct from one another.

3.2.1. Polypoidal choroidal vasculopathy (PCV)

PCV is considered to be a variant of AMD, and is characterized by abnormal choroidal vascular channels with terminal dilatations (the polyps), which are often seen as orange-red subretinal nodules (Fig. 6). ICGA is essential to the diagnosis of PCV.[9] While the criteria used to diagnose PCV in the literature are highly variable, some attempts at standardization of the diagnostic criteria have been made[9-11] and were used in the EVEREST study. The features of PCV on ICGA are the presence of an early area of hyperfluorescence (occurring within the first 5 minutes) which are associated with one of the following six criteria:

- A nodular appearance of the polyps on stereoscopic examination
- A dark (hypofluorescent) halo around the nodule
- Presence of a branching vascular network
- Pulsation of the nodule
- Orange-red subretinal nodules (on color fundus photography)
- Massive submacular hemorrhage (defined as an area of four disc areas or more on color fundus photography)

Both the presence of a branching vascular network and pulsation of the polyp can be visualized more clearly during the early phase of the angiogram, especially on dynamic video angiography using a CSLO device. Using these modalities, several subtypes of PCV have been described, with significant differences in long-term visual outcomes.[9]

3.2.2. Retinal angiomatous proliferation (RAP)

These lesions consist of neovascularization originating from the retina, which may anastomose with the choroidal circulation and can result in secondary CNV. ICGA allows visualization of the intraretinal vascular abnormalities and their circulation can be seen clearly on dynamic video angiography, originating from the arterioles and draining into a venule.

Three stages of RAP have been described:

- **Stage I — Intraretinal neovascularization**. The lesion is located within the retina, and manifests with an area of intense hyperfluorescence within the retina.
- **Stage II — Subretinal neovascularization**. The area of hyperfluorescence occurs within and beneath the retina.
- **Stage III — Choroidal neovascularization**. The presence of CNV is seen on both fluorescein and indocyanine green angiography.

More recently, based on OCT criteria, RAP has been re-labeled as Type 3 neovascularization.

3.2.3. Central serous chorioretinopathy

While the diagnosis of central serous chorioretinopathy can be made clinically and with fluorescein angiography, several diagnostic features can also be seen on indocyanine green angiography. Leakage points manifest with small hyperfluorescent spots which occur at the level of the retinal pigment epithelium (Fig. 3). These may persist and become more apparent during the later stages of the angiogram. Choroidal hyperpermeability manifests with areas of generalized hyperfluorescence, which obscures the outlines of the large choroidal vessels. This usually occurs within 5 to 10 minutes.

In cases of chronic or recurrent central serous chorioretinopathy, gravitational tracts can be seen due to tracking of the subretinal fluid inferiorly. These manifest as areas of hyper- or hypofluorescence which correspond to regions of retinal pigment epithelium atrophy.

3.2.4. Inflammatory eye diseases

In patients with active inflammation, lesions usually appear hypofluorescent due to masking of the choroidal fluorescence by the infiltrate, or due to areas of choroidal hypoperfusion. In later stages, these lesions may show some degree of staining.

4. Optical Coherence Tomography

4.1. *Principles of optical coherence tomography*

Optical Coherence Tomography (OCT) is a non-contact and non-invasive imaging technique that can produce high resolution cross-sectional images of the anterior segment of the eye, retina, retinal nerve fiber layer, optic nerve head and more recently, the choroid (Figs. 7–9).[12–16] It has been described as an "optical biopsy" of the eye.[16] OCT employs low-coherence interferometry to determine the echo time delay and magnitude of backscattered light from tissues. It illuminates the eye with light from a broadband source. Backscattered light is combined with that from the reference arm to generate an interferogram. In spectral domain OCT (SD-OCT), the signals are frequency encoded, and signals from greater depths have higher frequencies.[17] In contrast, for earlier time domain OCT (TD-OCT), the depth information is time delay encoded.

The first OCT devices introduced for clinical use were TD-OCT, such as the Stratus OCT (Carl Zeiss Meditec, Inc, Dublin, CA), which was introduced in 2002.[18] A typical TD-OCT has a scan speed of 400 A-scans per second and the B-scans have an axial resolution of about 10 μm.

SD-OCT became commercially available a few years later (Fig. 7). These commercial SD-OCT devices can achieve scan rates of over 70,000 A-scans per second and the B-scans have an axial resolution of 3–7 μm. The difference between TD- and SD-OCT lies in their respective mode of signal acquisition. Unlike the TD-OCT which uses an oscillating reference mirror to allow imaging of a known range of depths in the tissue, the SD-OCT's mirror is stationary. The inteferogram is split by a dispersive detector and the respective frequencies are simultaneously detected by a CCD. They then undergo a Fourier transformation and the scattering amplitude is obtained, thereby generating an *in vivo* depth profile of the tissue.[17] All points along each A-scan are gathered simultaneously and this greatly accelerates the scan speed.

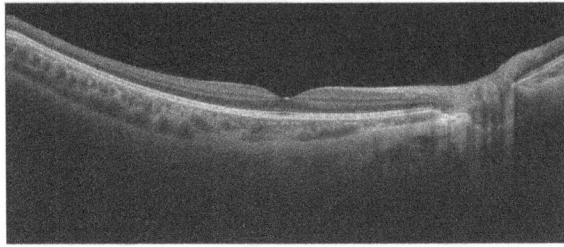

(A)

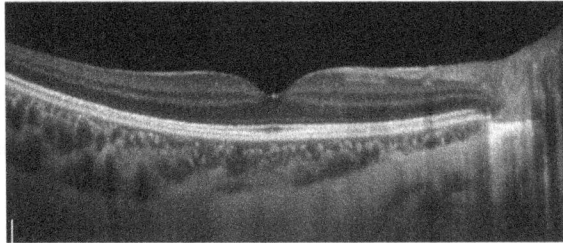

(B)

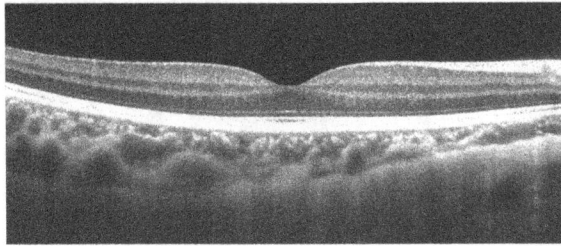

(C)

Figure 7. Optical coherence tomography (OCT) of a normal individual. (A) OCT from a swept source OCT device. (B & C) OCTs from spectral domain OCT devices.

Swept-source OCT (SS-OCT) is the latest milestone in retinal and choroidal imaging. The scan speed in SS-OCT can be considerably faster than that of SD-OCT, with scan rates of 100,000 A-scans/sec or more on commercial devices, with research prototype devices achieving speeds in the millions of A-scans/second. This faster B-scan acquisition allows for more dense and optimal three-dimensional imaging of the retina and choroid with higher degrees of averaging for improved image quality.[19] SS-OCT devices also feature light sources with a longer wavelength

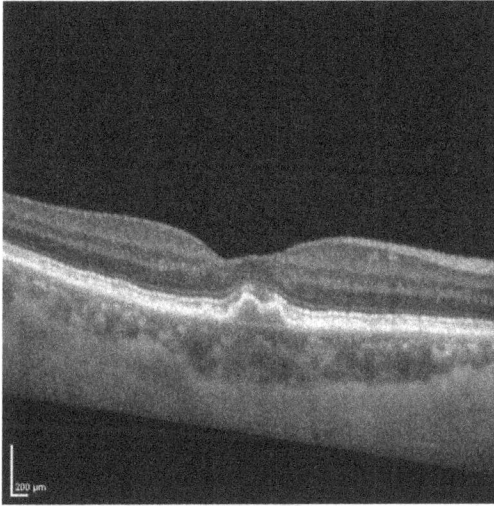

Figure 8. Optical coherence tomogram of drusen from a patient with non-neovascular age-related macular degeneration.

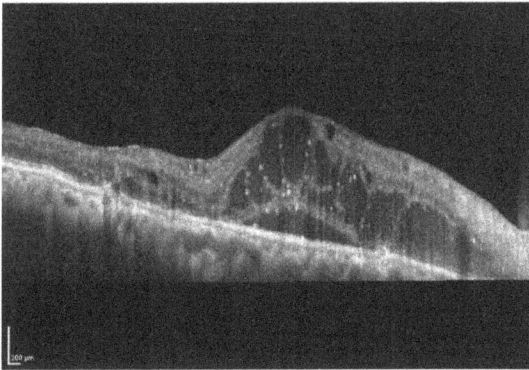

Figure 9. Optical coherence tomogram of a patient with diabetic macular edema. Intraretinal cysts with associated retinal thickening are seen. Subretinal fluid is present beneath the fovea.

(1050 nm, compared to 840 nm in SD-OCT) and photodetectors that produce less sensitivity roll-off, yielding less loss of signal with depth and better image quality for visualization of deeper structures such as the choroid.[20]

4.2. Choroidal imaging using OCT

Choroidal imaging is an area of considerable research interest in recent years and this is made possible by advances in OCT imaging.[16,21] While OCT has been used extensively to image the retina, RFNL and the optic nerve for more than a decade, the deeper layers, such as the choroid could not be adequately imaged with standard OCT due to: (1) Wavelength dependent light scattering (especially by the retinal pigment epithelium) and signal loss in the image path; (2) Decreasing sensitivity and resolution with increasing displacement from zero-delay; (3) Decreased maximal dynamic range inherent to Fourier domain systems; (4) lateral width of the defocused imaging beam; and (5) low signal-to-noise ratio of TD-OCT.[17,22]

SD-OCT can be used to image the choroid using techniques such as Enhanced Depth Imaging (EDI) and image averaging. EDI was first described by Spaide et al.[17] and involves pushing the OCT objective lens closer to the eye, such that an inverted image is obtained. As a result, the choroid and sclera are brought closer to the zero delay line, which improves resolution. Image averaging involves the acquisition of multiple B-scans from the same location which are then averaged together to increase the signal-to-noise ratio.[17]

Choroidal thickness can be measured using a line drawn perpendicularly from the hyperreflective line, which represents the retinal pigment epithelium (RPE), to the choroid–scleral junction using the proprietary software on most SD-OCT systems. Studies have established very good intraobserver, interobserver, and intrasession coefficients of repeatability.[23–27] A change of 32 μm was reported to likely exceed interobserver variability in subfoveal choroidal thickness.[23] Prototype software and even some current SS-OCT systems employ segmentation algorithms to measure choroidal thickness.

Mean subfoveal choroidal thickness is reported to range from 264.15 μm to 354 μm.[17,23–25,28–30] There is also significant topographic variation of choroidal thickness at different regions of the macula measured using OCT.[30] The choroid is reported to be thinnest nasally and relatively thick temporally.[30–32]

Diurnal variation in choroidal thickness is an essential consideration in studies of choroidal thickness.[33,34] In a paper published in 2012, Tan et al.[33]

demonstrated significant diurnal variation of choroidal thickness, with mean amplitude of 33.7 µm. The amplitude was significantly greater in choroids with thicker baseline choroidal thickness compared to the thinner choroids (43.1 vs. 10.5 µm, $p < 0.001$). The amplitude is also significantly correlated with age ($p = 0.032$), axial length ($p < 0.001$), spherical equivalent ($p < 0.001$) and change in systolic blood pressure ($p = 0.031$). Tracking and registration functionalities of the OCT device allow measurement of the same part of the choroid in between measurements to establish diurnal variation.

OCT systems are also used extensively to evaluate the choroid in many posterior segment diseases. In diseases such as AMD,[35,36] diabetic retinopathy,[37] retinal vein occlusion, pathologic myopia,[38,39] choroidal thickness has been found to be thinner compared to normal controls. In contrast, the choroid is significantly thickened in conditions such as central serous chorioretinopathy.[40,41] Variation in choroidal thickness may indicate the presence of a disease, demonstrate progression or recovery, and may provide information of prognostic value.

5. Fundus Autofluorescence

Autoflourescence is a phenomenon where tissues demonstrate fluorescence without the use of a dye (such as fluorescein). This occurs due to the presence of flurophores, an example of which is lipofuscin. Lipofuscin is produced as a by-product of photoreceptor shedding and is deposited in the lysosomes of retinal pigment epithelium cells following phagocytosis of the photoreceptor outer segments.[42-44] While lipofuscin is normally cleared by the retinal pigment epithelium, this process slows down over time due to normal ageing, especially in the presence of unhealthy or diseased retinal pigment epithelium cells. As a result, the concentration of lipofuscin increases, which results in greater autoflourescence from these tissues.[45]

Fundus autoflourescence is a non-invasive imaging method which detects autofluorescence from fluorophores in retinal tissues. Lipofuscin-derived fundus autoflourescence signals are emitted across a broad spectrum, ranging from 500 nm to 800 nm.[42] Consequently, it is possible to obtain fundus autofluorescence images using green (532 nm) and blue (488 nm) light.[44,45]

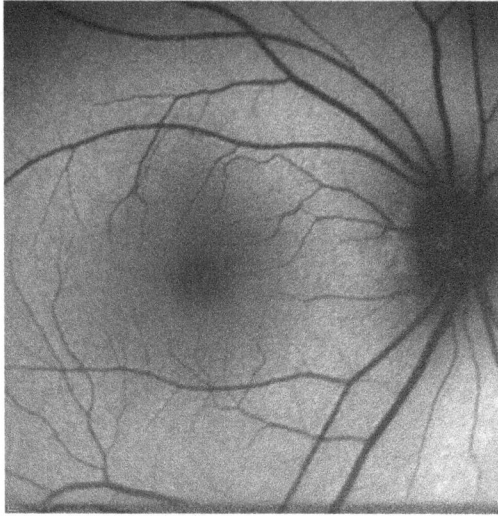

Figure 10.　Fundus autofluorescence from a normal individual. There is an area of hypo-autofluorescence at the fovea.

Fundus autofluorescence images can be captured using conventional fundus photography and confocal scanning laser ophthalmoscopy. Devices such as the Topcon TRC-50DX use flash photography with modified green-light filters (Spaide AF filters),[46] whereas the Heidleberg Spectralis devices use blue light to obtain the images.[45]

In clinical practice, fundus autofluorescence is commonly used to assess the health and function of the retinal pigment epithelium and the overlying neurosensory retina.[47,48] In a normal, healthy fundus, a typical fundus autofluorescence pattern is seen with reduced signal at the optic nerve head, retinal vessels and fovea, while the signal is slightly enhanced in the parafoveal region (Fig. 10). In the presence of retinal disease, the pattern of fundus autofluorescence changes. In regions with disease, lipofuscin accumulates in the retinal pigment epithelium, resulting in increased fundus autofluorescence. In contrast, in areas where the retinal pigment epithelium cells are very unhealthy or dead, such as in areas of retinal pigment epithelium atrophy, the lipofuscin content is reduced or absent, resulting in decreased fundus autofluorescence signals (Fig. 11).[49,50]

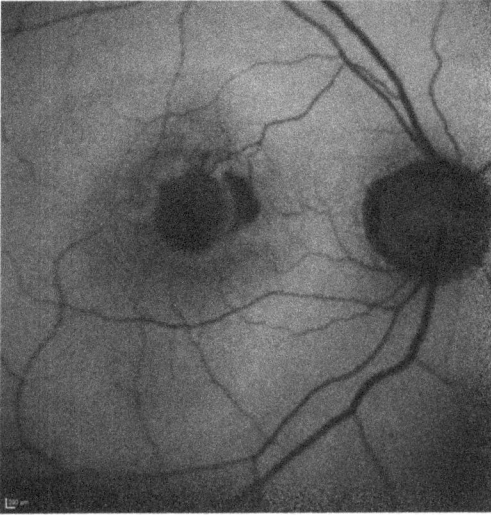

Figure 11. Fundus autofluorescence from a patient with geographic atrophy secondary to age-related macular degeneration. Two large areas of hypo-autofluorescence correspond to the geographic atrophy.

Fundus autofluorescence imaging plays important roles in detection of diseases, monitoring disease progress, prognosticating diseases, and providing functional correlation. In the assessment of retinal diseases, fundus autofluorescence can show the demarcation between healthy and viable retinal pigment epithelium cells and areas of geographic atrophy more distinctly than color fundus photography.[48,49] It can potentially demonstrate if the fovea has been involved, and hence aid the ophthalmologist in advising the patient on visual prognosis. When performed serially, it is possible to detect progression of the disease, as evident by an enlargement of the areas of decreased or absent fundus autofluorescence.[51] It has also been demonstrated that there is usually a ring of hyper autofluorescence around regions of decreased fundus autofluorescence, which indicate unhealthy tissue. These hyperautoflourescent regions are often the sites of progression of retinal pigment epithelium atrophy.[51,52]

Studies have characterized different patterns of abnormal fundus autofluorescence in the central 30 degrees of the macula.[48,53,54] It has been demonstrated that the various patterns are of prognostic significance, with some patterns such as the diffuse trickling pattern demonstrating higher rates of progression compared to others. More recently, studies using widefield imaging have also demonstrated distinct patterns of fundus autofluorescence changes in the periphery, with different frequencies of patterns among normal individuals and patients with neovascular and non-neovascular AMD.[55] This will be discussed in greater detail in the section on widefield imaging.

6. Widefield Imaging

The first commercially available fundus camera was produced by Carl Zeiss in 1926, providing a 20-degree field of view of the posterior pole. Subsequently, lenses covering between 30- to 55-degree fields of view became the standard for fundus imaging. It was recognized, however, that such images covered only a small proportion of the total retinal area, and attempts were made to obtain additional peripheral views to increase the coverage of the retina. The Early Treatment Diabetic Retinopathy Study (ETDRS) used a protocol which took stereo pair images in seven standard fields which, when viewed collectively, covered a 75-degree field of view.[56] This is still the current standard when conducting studies on diabetic retinopathy. Other studies such as the Central Vein Occlusion Study (CVOS)[57–59] and Branch Vein Occlusion Study (BVOS)[60,61] also utilized several fields of view to increase coverage of the posterior pole.

The Ocular Staurenghi 230 SLO Retina Lens (Ocular Instruments, Bellevue, Wash.) is a contact lens designed for use with a scanning laser ophthalmoscope. This consists of a separate handheld contact lens which needs to be applied to the eye prior to imaging, and is reported to produce an image with a 150-degree field of view.[62]

Heidelberg Engineering (Heidelberg, Germany) has recently introduced a non-contact ultra-widefield lens for use with the Spectralis Heidelberg Retinal Angiograph (HRA) system. This has been reported to produce high contrast evenly illuminated images of the peripheral retina and can be used for both fluorescein and indocyanine green angiography. The total retinal surface area imaged, however, is smaller than that produced by the Optos imaging systems.[63] In addition, the resolution is somewhat limited.

Optos (Dunfermline, Scotland) has produced a series of instruments such as the Optos 200Tx for ultra-widefield imaging. The Optos system features an ellipsoid mirror to create a focal point within the eye, without the need for a contact lens or pupil dilation.[64,65] By using a scanning laser ophthalmoscope, there is no need for a bright flash illumination. The Optos 200Tx is able to produce pseudo-color images (resolution 20 μm), fluorescein angiograms (resolution 14 μm), autofluorescence and ResMax images (covering 100 degrees, with a higher resolution of 11 μm). The ultra-widefield images cover up to a 200-degree internal field of view, which is estimated to be 82.5% of the total retinal surface area. Ultra-widefield images produced by this device do not image the superior and inferior periphery as well compared to the nasal and temporal regions, without steering the images in these vertical directions. Another limitation of this (and all widefield imaging systems, for that matter) is the warping of the images at the periphery. However, software has recently become available that creates a more anatomically correct stereographic projection image, allowing precise measurements to be made on widefield images.

The RetCam (Clarity Medical Systems, Pleasanton, CA, USA) is a widefield digital imaging system designed to produce color and fluorescein angiogram images covering an angle of up to 120 degrees. This can be used in the clinic, operating room or neonatal wards. It is useful for objective documentation of findings, and allows serial comparisons during the course of follow-up. The ability to transmit digital images is also useful for remote tele-ophthalmology screening and diagnosis.

The Panoret-1000 (CMT Medical Technologies Inc., Valley Stream, NY) is a portable device which can image 130 degrees of the fundus. This device differs from the others in that it employs transscleral rather than transpupillary illumination.

6.1. *Pseudocolor fundus images*

Widefield pseudocolor fundus images have been shown to detect a higher proportion of peripheral retinal pathology compared to conventional imaging, especially for lesions which are commonly located more peripherally, such as retinal holes and tears. It has also been shown to be of importance in screening for diabetic retinopathy and retinopathy of prematurity, and the detection and monitoring of ocular tumors and cytomegalovirus retinitis. Several studies comparing widefield color fundus photography with ETDRS 7-field imaging and dilated fundal examination have reported good comparability of the various modalities in the classification of diabetic retinopathy.[66-69] A recent study by Silva et al.[67] reported that the diabetic retinopathy severity between widefield imaging and ETDRS photography matched in 80% of eyes, and was within one level in 94.5% of eyes (weighted kappa 0.74). Widefield imaging has the additional advantage of faster acquisition time (a single image compared to seven stereo-pair images for the ETDRS protocol) and for imaging through small apertures (e.g. undilated pupils, or small openings in significant cataracts). The study further reported that 20% of eyes had discrepancies between widefield fundus photographs and ETDRS photographs, with approximately one-third of hemorrhages/ microaneurysms, intraretinal microvascular abnormalities and new-vessels elsewhere occurring predominantly outside the ETDRS fields. This resulted in a more severe assessment of DR in 10% of eyes compared to the grading based on ETDRS fields,[67] although the clinical significance of these findings remain uncertain.

An important application of the RetCam is for screening and monitoring of progression of retinopathy of prematurity (ROP). Various studies have reported high sensitivities and specificities when the RetCam is used for retinopathy of prematurity screening. In a review of seven Level I and three level III studies published in 2012, Chiang et al.[70] concluded that digital retinal photography has high accuracy for detection of clinically significant retinopathy of prematurity.

6.2. Widefield fluorescein angiography

Widefield imaging devices can be used to capture fluorescein angiograms of the periphery, which allows detection of peripheral ischemia[71-75] and peripheral leakage from uveitis. Recent studies have shown that patients with retinal vascular diseases such as diabetic retinopathy and retinal vein occlusion manifest with areas of non-perfusion which lie outside the zone imaged by conventional fluorescein angiograms. A study by Wessel et al.[76] reported that widefield fluorescein angiography revealed up to 3.9 times more non-perfusion compared to ETDRS fields, including

1.9 times more new vessels elsewhere. This has led to interest in targeted photocoagulation[77] based on the areas of non-perfusion detected, rather than pan-retinal photocoagulation, though prospective studies confirming the validity of this approach have not yet been reported.

It has been shown that the presence and extent of peripheral non-perfusion correlates with the presence and severity of diabetic macular edema and its response to treatment. Wessel *et al.*[71] reported a significant correlation between the presence of diabetic macular edema and peripheral ischemia, and that patients with peripheral non-perfusion had a 3.75 times greater odds of having diabetic macular edema compared to those without non-perfusion. Similar results have also been reported in studies on retinal vein occlusion. In a study by Singer *et al.*,[73] patients having larger areas of non-perfusion at baseline manifested with greater retinal thickening and poorer visual acuity compared to those with smaller areas. These findings have led investigators to suggest that the extent of peripheral non-perfusion may influence the release of VEGF, which in turn causes macular edema.

6.3. Widefield fundus autofluorescence

The Optos 200Tx has been adapted to produce green-light (532 nm) fundus autofluorescence images, and has been shown to be of value in diseases such as AMD, hereditary fundus dystrophies, and inflammatory conditions. In a study of 470 eyes of 248 patients seen in a tertiary retinal clinic, FAF abnormalities were detected in 65.5% of eyes.[78] The frequency of peripheral FAF abnormalities varied with the type of disease, being highest among patients with retinal dystrophies (82.2%), AMD (73.9%), ocular tumors (72.7%), and inflammatory conditions (68.5%).

Although AMD has been considered to be primarily a macular disease, studies have shown that peripheral FAF abnormalities are present in patients with AMD. In a study involving 105 patients with AMD and 19 normal controls, 68.9% of eyes had distinct FAF abnormalities, with higher frequency among those with neovascular AMD compared to non-neovascular AMD and normal eyes (86% vs. 72.8% vs. 18.4% respectively).[55] The significant risk factors for the presence of peripheral FAF abnormalities included the AMD type, older age, and female sex. It was also reported that the patterns of peripheral FAF abnormalities correlated well with clinical features seen on widefield color photographs.[55]

A study by Oishi[79] of 75 patients with retinitis pigmentosa reported that the type and extent of FAF abnormalities can be used to estimate the duration of disease and the visual field pattern. Patients without hyperautofluorescent rings or foveal hyperautofluorescence had better visual acuity and mean deviation on Humphrey visual fields. Patients with large patchy hypofluorescent areas were older than those with small areas, and had experienced symptoms for longer durations.

7. Conclusion

In this chapter, we have provided an overview of the imaging modalities commonly used for the posterior pole, and the characteristic features of common retinal diseases, although it is not possible to cover all diseases in this short space. It is important for ophthalmologists to recognize the relative strengths and weaknesses of each modality, so that the appropriate investigation can be utilized. It is also helpful to view these modalities as complementary to one another, with each providing a broad array of information on the patient's condition.

8. References

1. Subfoveal neovascular lesions in age-related macular degeneration. Guidelines for evaluation and treatment in the macular photocoagulation study. Macular Photocoagulation Study Group. *Arch Ophthalmol* **109**, 1242–1257 (1991).
2. Photodynamic therapy of subfoveal choroidal neovascularization in age-related macular degeneration with verteporfin: one-year results of 2 randomized clinical trials — TAP report. Treatment of age-related macular degeneration with photodynamic therapy (TAP) Study Group. *Arch Ophthalmol* **117**, 1329–1345 (1999).
3. Guidelines for using verteporfin (visudyne) in photodynamic therapy to treat choroidal neovascularization due to age-related macular degeneration and other causes. *Retina* **22**, 6–18 (2002).
4. Barbazetto, I., Burdan, A., Bressler, N.M., *et al.* Photodynamic therapy of subfoveal choroidal neovascularization with verteporfin: fluorescein angiographic

guidelines for evaluation and treatment — TAP and VIP report No. 2. *Arch Ophthalmol* **121**, 1253–1268 (2003).

5. Watzke, R.C., Klein, M.L., Hiner, C.J., *et al.* A comparison of stereoscopic fluorescein angiography with indocyanine green videoangiography in age-related macular degeneration. *Ophthalmology* **107**, 1601–1606 (2000).

6. Hariri, A., Heussen, F.M., Nittala, M.G., Sadda, S.R. Optical coherence tomographic correlates of angiographic subtypes of occult choroidal neovascularization. *Invest Ophthalmol Vis Sci* **54**, 8020–8026 (2013).

7. Yannuzzi, L.A, Hope-Ross, M., Slakter, J.S., *et al.* Analysis of vascularized pigment epithelial detachments using indocyanine green videoangiography. *Retina* **14**, 99–113 (1994).

8. Guyer, D.R., Yannuzzi, L.A., Slakter, J.S., *et al.* Classification of choroidal neovascularization by digital indocyanine green videoangiography. *Ophthalmology* **103**, 2054–2060 (1996).

9. Tan, C.S., Ngo, W.K., Lim, L.W., Lim, T.H. A novel classification of the vascular patterns of polypoidal choroidal vasculopathy and its relation to clinical outcomes. *Br J Ophthalmol* (2014).

10. Lim, T.H., Laude, A., Tan, C.S. Polypoidal choroidal vasculopathy: an angiographic discussion. *Eye (Lond)* **24**, 483–490 (2010).

11. Tan, C.S., Wong, H.T., Lim, B.A., *et al.* Polypoidal choroidal vasculopathy causing massive suprachoroidal haemorrhage. *Eye (Lond)* **21**, 132–133 (2007).

12. Huang, D., Swanson, E.A., Lin, C.P., *et al.* Optical coherence tomography. *Science* **254**, 1178–1181 (1991).

13. Hee, M.R., Izatt, J.A., Swanson, E.A., *et al.* Optical coherence tomography of the human retina. *Arch Ophthalmol* **113**, 325–332 (1995).

14. Puliafito, C.A., Hee, M.R., Lin, C.P., *et al.* Imaging of macular diseases with optical coherence tomography. *Ophthalmology* **102**, 217–229 (1995).

15. Hee, M.R., Puliafito, C.A., Wong, C., *et al.* Quantitative assessment of macular edema with optical coherence tomography. *Arch Ophthalmol* **113**, 1019–1029 (1995).

16. Adhi, M., Duker, J.S. Optical coherence tomography — current and future applications. *Curr Opin Ophthalmol* **24**, 213–221 (2013).

17. Spaide, R.F., Koizumi, H., Pozzoni, M.C. Enhanced depth imaging spectral-domain optical coherence tomography. *Am J Ophthalmol* **146**, 496–500 (2008).

18. Sull, A.C., Vuong, L.N., Price, L.L., *et al.* Comparison of spectral/Fourier domain optical coherence tomography instruments for assessment of normal macular thickness. *Retina* **30**, 235–245 (2010).

19. Adhi, M., Liu, J.J., Qavi, A.H., et al. Enhanced visualization of the choroido-scleral interface using swept-source OCT. Ophthalmic Surg Lasers Imaging Retina **44**, S40–S42 (2013).
20. Mrejen, S., Spaide, R.F. Optical coherence tomography: imaging of the choroid and beyond. Surv Ophthalmol **58**, 387–429 (2013).
21. Wong, I.Y., Koizumi, H., Lai, W.W. Enhanced depth imaging optical coherence tomography. Ophthalmic Surg Lasers Imaging **42**, S75–S84 (2011).
22. Spaide, R.F. Enhanced depth imaging optical coherence tomography of retinal pigment epithelial detachment in age-related macular degeneration. Am J Ophthalmol **147**, 644–652 (2009).
23. Rahman, W., Chen, F.K., Yeoh, J., et al. Repeatability of manual subfoveal choroidal thickness measurements in healthy subjects using the technique of enhanced depth imaging optical coherence tomography. Invest Ophthalmol Vis Sci **52**, 2267–2271 (2011).
24. Ikuno, Y., Maruko, I., Yasuno, Y., et al. Reproducibility of retinal and choroidal thickness measurements in enhanced depth imaging and high-penetration optical coherence tomography. Invest Ophthalmol Vis Sci **52**, 5536–5540 (2011).
25. Chhablani, J., Barteselli, G., Wang, H., et al. Repeatability and reproducibility of manual choroidal volume measurements using enhanced depth imaging optical coherence tomography. Invest Ophthalmol Vis Sci **53**, 2274–2280 (2012).
26. Shao, L., Xu, L., Chen, C.X., et al. Reproducibility of subfoveal choroidal thickness measurements with enhanced depth imaging by spectral-domain optical coherence tomography. Invest Ophthalmol Vis Sci **54**, 230–233 (2013).
27. Branchini, L., Regatieri, C.V., Flores-Moreno, I., et al. Reproducibility of choroidal thickness measurements across three spectral domain optical coherence tomography systems. Ophthalmology **119**, 119–123 (2012).
28. Margolis, R., Spaide, R.F. A pilot study of enhanced depth imaging optical coherence tomography of the choroid in normal eyes. Am J Ophthalmol **147**, 811–815 (2009).
29. Ikuno, Y., Kawaguchi, K., Nouchi, T., Yasuno, Y. Choroidal thickness in healthy Japanese subjects. Invest Ophthalmol Vis Sci **51**, 2173–2176 (2010).
30. Tan, C.S., Cheong, K.X., Lim, L.W., Li, K.Z. Topographic variation of choroidal and retinal thicknesses at the macula in healthy adults. Br J Ophthalmol **98**, 339–344 (2014).
31. Agawa, T., Miura, M., Ikuno, Y., et al. Choroidal thickness measurement in healthy Japanese subjects by three-dimensional high-penetration optical coherence tomography. Graefes Arch Clin Exp Ophthalmol **249**, 1485–1492 (2011).

32. Tanabe, H., Ito, Y., Terasaki, H. Choroid is thinner in inferior region of optic disks of normal eyes. *Retina* **32**, 134–139 (2012).

33. Tan, C.S., Ouyang, Y., Ruiz, H., Sadda, S.R. Diurnal variation of choroidal thickness in normal, healthy subjects measured by spectral domain optical coherence tomography. *Invest Ophthalmol Vis Sci* **53**, 261–266 (2012).

34. Usui, S., Ikuno, Y., Akiba, M., *et al.* Circadian changes in subfoveal choroidal thickness and the relationship with circulatory factors in healthy subjects. *Invest Ophthalmol Vis Sci* **53**, 2300–2307 (2012).

35. Manjunath, V., Goren, J., Fujimoto, J.G., Duker, J.S. Analysis of choroidal thickness in age-related macular degeneration using spectral-domain optical coherence tomography. *Am J Ophthalmol* **152**, 663–668 (2011).

36. Chung, S.E., Kang, S.W., Lee, J.H., Kim, Y.T. Choroidal thickness in polypoidal choroidal vasculopathy and exudative age-related macular degeneration. *Ophthalmology* **118**, 840–845 (2011).

37. Regatieri, C.V., Branchini, L., Carmody, J., *et al.* Choroidal thickness in patients with diabetic retinopathy analyzed by spectral-domain optical coherence tomography. *Retina* **32**, 563–568 (2012).

38. Ikuno, Y., Tano, Y. Retinal and choroidal biometry in highly myopic eyes with spectral-domain optical coherence tomography. *Invest Ophthalmol Vis Sci* **50**, 3876–3880 (2009).

39. Coscas, G., Zhou, Q., Coscas, F., *et al.* Choroid thickness measurement with RTVue optical coherence tomography in emmetropic eyes, mildly myopic eyes, and highly myopic eyes. *Eur J Ophthalmol* **22**, 992–1000 (2012).

40. Maruko, I., Iida, T., Sugano, Y., *et al.* Subfoveal choroidal thickness in fellow eyes of patients with central serous chorioretinopathy. *Retina* **31**, 1603–1608 (2011).

41. Pryds, A., Larsen, M. Choroidal thickness following extrafoveal photodynamic treatment with verteporfin in patients with central serous chorioretinopathy. *Acta Ophthalmol* **90**, 738–743 (2012).

42. Delori, F.C., Dorey, C.K., Staurenghi, G., *et al. In vivo* fluorescence of the ocular fundus exhibits retinal pigment epithelium lipofuscin characteristics. *Invest Ophthalmol Vis Sci* **36**, 718–729 (1995).

43. Sparrow, J.R., Boulton, M. RPE lipofuscin and its role in retinal pathobiology. *Exp Eye Res* **80**, 595–606 (2005).

44. Sparrow, J.R., Yoon, K.D., Wu, Y., Yamamoto, K. Interpretations of fundus autofluorescence from studies of the bisretinoids of the retina. *Invest Ophthalmol Vis Sci* **51**, 4351–4357 (2010).

45. Wolf-Schnurrbusch, U.E., Wittwer, V.V., Ghanem, R., *et al.* Blue-light versus green-light autofluorescence: lesion size of areas of geographic atrophy. *Invest Ophthalmol Vis Sci* **52**, 9497–9502 (2011).

46. Spaide, R.F. Fundus autofluorescence and age-related macular degeneration. *Ophthalmology* **110**, 392–399 (2003).

47. Delori, F.C., Fleckner, M.R., Goger, D.G., *et al.* Autofluorescence distribution associated with drusen in age-related macular degeneration. *Invest Ophthalmol Vis Sci* **41**, 496–504 (2000).

48. Bindewald, A., Bird, A.C., Dandekar, S.S., *et al.* Classification of fundus autofluorescence patterns in early age-related macular disease. *Invest Ophthalmol Vis Sci* **46**, 3309–3314 (2005).

49. Schmitz-Valckenberg, S., Holz, F.G., Bird, A.C., Spaide, R.F. Fundus autofluorescence imaging: review and perspectives. *Retina* **28**, 385–409 (2008).

50. Sepah, Y.J., Akhtar, A., Sadiq, M.A., *et al.* Fundus autofluorescence imaging: Fundamentals and clinical relevance. *Saudi J Ophthalmol* **28**, 111–116 (2014).

51. von, R.A., Fitzke, F.W., Bird, A.C. Fundus autofluorescence in age-related macular disease imaged with a laser scanning ophthalmoscope. *Invest Ophthalmol Vis Sci* **38**, 478–486 (1997).

52. Holz, F.G., Bellman, C., Staudt, S., *et al.* Fundus autofluorescence and development of geographic atrophy in age-related macular degeneration. *Invest Ophthalmol Vis Sci* **42**, 1051–1056 (2001).

53. Holz, F.G., Bellmann, C., Margaritidis, M., *et al.* Patterns of increased *in vivo* fundus autofluorescence in the junctional zone of geographic atrophy of the retinal pigment epithelium associated with age-related macular degeneration. *Graefes Arch Clin Exp Ophthalmol* **237**, 145–152 (1999).

54. Holz, F.G., Bindewald-Wittich, A., Fleckenstein, M., *et al.* Progression of geographic atrophy and impact of fundus autofluorescence patterns in age-related macular degeneration. *Am J Ophthalmol* **143**, 463–472 (2007).

55. Tan, C.S., Heussen, F., Sadda, S.R. Peripheral autofluorescence and clinical findings in neovascular and non-neovascular age-related macular degeneration. *Ophthalmology* **120**, 1271–1277 (2013).

56. Diabetic retinopathy study. Report Number 6. Design, methods, and baseline results. Report Number 7. A modification of the Airlie House classification of diabetic retinopathy. Prepared by the Diabetic Retinopathy. *Invest Ophthalmol Vis Sci* **21**, 1–226 (1981).

57. Evaluation of grid pattern photocoagulation for macular edema in central vein occlusion. The Central Vein Occlusion Study Group M report. *Ophthalmology* **102**, 1425–1433 (1995).

58. A randomized clinical trial of early panretinal photocoagulation for ischemic central vein occlusion. The Central Vein Occlusion Study Group N report. *Ophthalmology* **102**, 1434–1444 (1995).

59. Natural history and clinical management of central retinal vein occlusion. The Central Vein Occlusion Study Group. *Arch Ophthalmol* **115**, 486–491 (1997).

60. Argon laser scatter photocoagulation for prevention of neovascularization and vitreous hemorrhage in branch vein occlusion. A randomized clinical trial. Branch Vein Occlusion Study Group. *Arch Ophthalmol* **104**, 34–41 (1986).

61. Argon laser photocoagulation for macular edema in branch vein occlusion. The Branch Vein Occlusion Study Group. *Am J Ophthalmol* **98**, 271–282 (1984).

62. Staurenghi, G., Viola, F., Mainster, M.A., *et al.* Scanning laser ophthalmoscopy and angiography with a wide-field contact lens system. *Arch Ophthalmol* **123**, 244–252 (2005).

63. Witmer, M.T., Parlitsis, G., Patel, S., Kiss, S. Comparison of ultra-widefield fluorescein angiography with the Heidelberg Spectralis((R)) noncontact ultra-widefield module versus the Optos((R)) Optomap((R)). *Clin Ophthalmol* **7**, 389–394 (2013).

64. Friberg, T.R., Gupta, A., Yu, J., *et al.* Ultrawide angle fluorescein angiographic imaging: a comparison to conventional digital acquisition systems. *Ophthalmic Surg Lasers Imaging* **39**, 304–311 (2008).

65. Spaide, R.F. Peripheral areas of nonperfusion in treated central retinal vein occlusion as imaged by wide-field fluorescein angiography. *Retina* **31**, 829–837 (2011).

66. Silva, P.S., Cavallerano, J.D,. Sun, J.K., *et al.* Nonmydriatic ultrawide field retinal imaging compared with dilated standard 7-field 35-mm photography and retinal specialist examination for evaluation of diabetic retinopathy. *Am J Ophthalmol* **154**, 549–559 (2012).

67. Silva, P.S., Cavallerano, J.D., Sun, J.K., *et al.* Peripheral lesions identified by mydriatic ultrawide field imaging: distribution and potential impact on diabetic retinopathy severity. *Ophthalmology* **120**, 2587–2595 (2013).

68. Kernt, M., Hadi, I., Pinter, F., *et al.* Assessment of diabetic retinopathy using nonmydriatic ultra-widefield scanning laser ophthalmoscopy (Optomap) compared with ETDRS 7-field stereo photography. *Diabetes Care* **35**, 2459–2463 (2012).

69. Soliman, A.Z., Silva, P.S., Aiello, L.P., Sun, J.K. Ultra-wide field retinal imaging in detection, classification, and management of diabetic retinopathy. *Semin Ophthalmol* **27**, 221–227 (2012).

70. Chiang, M.F., Melia, M., Buffenn, A.N., *et al.* Detection of clinically significant retinopathy of prematurity using wide-angle digital retinal photography: a report by the American Academy of Ophthalmology. *Ophthalmology* **119**, 1272–1280 (2012).

71. Wessel, M.M., Nair, N., Aaker, G.D., *et al.* Peripheral retinal ischaemia, as evaluated by ultra-widefield fluorescein angiography, is associated with diabetic macular oedema. *Br J Ophthalmol* **96**, 694–698 (2012).

72. Oliver, S.C., Schwartz, S.D. Peripheral vessel leakage (PVL): a new angiographic finding in diabetic retinopathy identified with ultra wide-field fluorescein angiography. *Semin Ophthalmol* **25**, 27–33 (2010).

73. Singer, M., Tan, C.S., Bell, D., Sadda, S.R. Area of peripheral retinal nonperfusion and treatment response in branch and central retinal vein occlusion. *Retina* (2014).

74. Tsui, I., Kaines, A., Havunjian, M.A., *et al.* Ischemic index and neovascularization in central retinal vein occlusion. *Retina* **31**, 105–110 (2011).

75. Prasad, P.S., Oliver, S.C., Coffee, R.E., *et al.* Ultra wide-field angiographic characteristics of branch retinal and hemicentral retinal vein occlusion. *Ophthalmology* **117**, 780–784 (2010).

76. Wessel, M.M., Aaker, G.D., Parlitsis, G., *et al.* Ultra-wide-field angiography improves the detection and classification of diabetic retinopathy. *Retina* **32**, 785–791 (2012).

77. Reddy, S., Hu, A., Schwartz, S.D. Ultra wide field fluorescein angiography guided targeted retinal photocoagulation (TRP). *Semin Ophthalmol* **24**, 9–14 (2009).

78. Heussen, F.M., Tan, C.S., Sadda, S.R. Prevalence of peripheral abnormalities on ultra-widefield greenlight (532 nm) autofluorescence imaging at a tertiary care center. *Invest Ophthalmol Vis Sci* **53**, 6526–6531 (2012).

79. Oishi, A., Ogino, K., Makiyama, Y., *et al.* Wide-field fundus autofluorescence imaging of retinitis pigmentosa. *Ophthalmology* **120**, 1827–1834 (2013).

Chapter 3: Pharmacogenomics of Response to Anti-VEGF Therapy in Exudative Age-Related Macular Degeneration

Seanna Grob,* Kang Zhang[†] and Sophie J. Bakri[‡]

*Massachusetts Eye and Ear Infirmary,
Harvard Medical School, Boston, MA
[†]Shiley Eye Institute, University of California San Diego,
La Jolla, CA
[‡]Department of Ophthalmology, Mayo Clinic, Rochester, MN

1. Introduction

Neovascular ("wet") age-related macular degeneration (AMD), a leading cause of blindness, is a pathologic age-related condition of the macula that causes severe impairment of vision in people aged over 50.[1] Neovascular AMD is characterized by central vision loss due to exudation, hemorrhage, and fibrovascular tissue formation secondary to pathologic choroidal neovascularization (CNV).[2] Factors presumed to be involved in the pathogenesis of CNV include ischemia, inflammation and the secretion of angiogenic factors, such as vascular endothelial growth factor (VEGF).[1]

VEGF is a homodimeric glycoprotein isolated from CNV membranes obtained from patients with AMD. It is a key regulator of physiologic and pathologic angiogenesis and a potent vascular permeability factor, increasing fluid leakage across blood vessel walls.[1,3] As studies have confirmed the necessity of VEGF (specifically VEGF-A in intraocular tissue) for the induction of neovascularization, it has emerged as a target for anti-angiogenic intravitreal medications for the treatment of CNV in AMD.[1] The anti-VEGF agents currently employed in the treatment of CNV include monoclonal antibodies, such as ranibizumab and bevacizumab, and fusion proteins, such as aflibercept, that antagonize the activity of

63

VEGF-A.[1,4] Numerous trials (MARINA, PrONTO, HARBOR, VIEW 1, VIEW 2, CATT and IVAN) have examined the efficacy and safety of various intravitreal anti-VEGF therapies, namely ranibizumab and bevacizumab.[4,5] While no universal consensus has been established for the optimal treatment and dosing regimen of these medications, they may be administered as often as monthly.[4]

While the emergence of anti-VEGF therapies has revolutionized the treatment of neovascular AMD, not all patients treated with these medications are equally responsive.[6] There are various definitions of which patients constitute "responders" and "non-responders". Some define treatment success as stabilization of vision (within three lines) loss while others focus on visual acuity (VA) gains and decrease in fluid on optical coherence tomography (OCT).[7] In patients deemed non-responders or suboptimal responders, genetic variations may be to blame. Recently, an association between genotype and response to supplementation with antioxidants and zinc (AREDS supplementation) was demonstrated.[30] Patients with no risk-alleles of complement factor H (CFH) and with one or two risk-alleles of age-related maculopathy susceptibility 2 (ARMS2 or LOC387715) derived the most benefit from zinc-only supplementation, whereas patients with one or two risk-alleles of CFH and no risk-alleles of ARMS2 derived the most benefit from antioxidant-only supplementation and had increased progression to advanced AMD with zinc supplementation.[30] This data suggests that genotype may influence response to therapy for AMD and that personalization of therapy may result in better outcomes.

Developments in genetic research of AMD have led to the identification of single nucleotide polymorphisms (SNPs) in multiple genes associated with various stages of AMD and/or risk or protective factors. Genome-wide association studies (GWAS) have led to the identification of the Y402H (rs1061170) variant within the CFH gene on chromosome 1q31, and has replicated the findings of the involvement of other genes implicated in AMD, ARMS2 and high-temperature requirement factor A1 (HTRA1), both on chromosome 10q26.[8–10]

In the CFH gene variation, a tyrosine-to-histidine substitution occurs at the amino acid position 402 (Y402H) as a result of a thymine-to-cytosine transition in exon 9 of the gene.[11,12] For the CFH Y402H polymorphism, the risk-allele is C (homozygous CC) and the heterozygote variant is TC. An alanine-to-serine substitution in codon 69 (A69S) has been found within the ARMS2 gene and the HTRA1 gene variations result from alterations in the GC-rich promoter sequence.[11,12] For the ARMS2 polymorphism, the homozygote for the risk-allele is TT and the heterozygote variant is GT; for the HTRA1 polymorphism, the risk-allele is A and the heterozygote variant is GA.[12] In the complement component 3 (C3) genetic variants, a glycine-to-arginine substitution occurs in codon 80 (R80G).[11] Variants in other genes implicated in the development of AMD include the apolipoprotein E (APOE) gene and the VEGF gene, both involved in angiogenesis and neovascularization.[13]

As variations in treatment have been found and certain genes have been associated with AMD, it has been hypothesized that genetic background may influence an individual's response to treatment. While some studies have found associations between certain SNPs and poor response to intravitreal anti-VEGF therapy for neovascular AMD, other studies have not corroborated these findings. This review summarizes the studies to date in this area (Table 1).

2. Results

2.1. *Pharmacogenetics for genes associated with AMD in the comparison of AMD treatments trials (CATT)*

The CATT was a large, 1-year, multicenter, single-masked, randomized, prospective, non-inferiority trial involving patients with treatment-naïve neovascular AMD. Patients were randomized to receive intravitreal injections of ranibizumab or bevacizumab every 4 weeks (q4wk) or prn after the first injection with a q4wk evaluation. After 52 weeks, a second randomization to either continue q4wk dosing or switch to as needed or prn treatment was performed for patients initially assigned to the q4wk dosing regimen. OCT was performed at every follow-up visit. Patients on the prn treatment regimen received intravitreal injections if fluid was present on OCT. Peripheral blood was collected from each patient and the following four AMD-associated SNPs were evaluated: (1) CFH (rs1061170); (2) ARMS2 (rs10490924); (3) HTRA1 (rs11200638); and (4) C3

Table 1. Summary of studies on genetic background and response to anti-VEGF treatment for neovascular AMD.

Study	Treatment	Genes	Non-responder Criteria	Frequency of Injections	Results	Limitations
Hagstrom SA[11]	Ranibizumab or bevacizumab	CFH [rs1061170], ARMS2 [rs10490924], HTRA1 [rs11200638], C3 [rs2230199]	VA worsened from baseline	q4w vs. prn (7–8/1 year)**	No association with VA outcomes, anatomic outcomes or the number of injections	• Combined results for both treatments reported only
Lee AY[14]	Ranibizumab	CFH [rs1061170]	—	3.3–3.9/9 months	CHF TC and CC are associated with an increased number of injections and decreased interval between injections	• Retrospective • Inconsistent follow-up with different cohorts • prn treatment regimen
Nischler C[15]	Bevacizumab	CFH [rs1061170]	Loss of ≥3 lines of VA	3.75/11.3 months (mean)	CHF CC is associated with worse VA outcomes; no association between genotype and type of CNV lesion	• Small • prn treatment regimen
Brantley MA[16]	Bevacizumab	CFH [rs1061170], ARMS2 [rs10490924]	No improvement in VA	prn (0.27–0.332/1 year)	CFH TT and TC and ARMS2 GG and GT with greater improvement in VA	• Small • Retrospective • No consideration of smoking status • prn treatment regiment

Study	Drug	Genes [SNPs]	Outcome measure	Follow-up	Findings	Limitations
Teper SJ[12]	Ranibizumab	CFH [rs1061170], ARMS2 [rs10490924]	—	5.77 ± 1.51/1 year#	CFH TT and TC with greater improvement in VA	• Small • Not all patients were treatment-naïve • No consideration of smoking status • prn treatment regimen
Orlin A[17]	Ranibizumab and/or bevacizumab	CFH [rs1061170], ARMS2 [rs10490924, rs3750848, del443ins54], HTRA1 [rs11200638, rs932275]	Decrease in VA from baseline or final VA <20/200	9.8 ± 0.62 and 10.26 ± 0.84/24 and 22 months (non-responders and responders)#	No associations observed	• Retrospective • Arbitrary criteria for definition of responder vs. non-responder • No consideration of smoking status • prn treatment regimen
McKibbin M[13]	Ranibizumab	CFH [rs1061170], VEGF [rs1413711], HRTA1 [rs11200638]	Loss of ≥15 ETDRS letters	3.7–4.2/6 months#	CFH and VEGF high-risk homozygous with more favorable VA outcome, not significant	• Small • Retrospective • Short follow-up period • prn treatment regimen

(Continued)

S. Grob, K. Zhang and S. J. Bakri

Table 1. (*Continued*)

Study	Treatment	Genes	Non-responder criteria	Frequency of injections	Results	Limitations
Tian J[18]	Bevacizumab	CFH [rs800292, rs1061170, rs10801555, rs1410996], ARMS2 [rs10490924], HTRA1 [rs11200638], VEGF [rs833069, rs3025039], SERPING1 [rs1005510, rs2511989], C3 [rs2230205, rs2250656]	—	3/12 weeks#	CFH [rs800292] TT, ARMS2 [rs10490924] TG and HTRA1 heterozygote with greatest improvement in VA	• Short follow-up period • Treatment at 6 week intervals vs. 4 week intervals
Lazzeri A[19]	Ranibizumab	VEGF-A [rs699947, rs1570360]	—	3/8 weeks#	VEGF-A [rs699947] wild-type variant with worse visual outcome	• Small • Short follow-up period • Exclusion of patients with predominantly hemorrhagic lesions • No consideration of smoking status

Francis PJ[20]	Ranibizumab	CFH [rs1065489, rs3753394, rs3766404], ARMS2 [rs10490924], C3 [rs1389623, rs2230205], VEGF-A [rs3025033, rs833069, rs833068], CTGF [rs9399005], FLT1 [rs9319428, rs9319425, rs622227, rs2387632, rs10507386, rs615529, rs7995976], THBS1 [rs1478604], FGFR2 [rs1047100, rs2912762] and others	—	7/1 year	Minor allele associations: CFH [rs1065489] and CTGF with worse VA; C3 [rs2230205] with greater reduction in retinal thickness; CFH with greater number of injections and VEGF-A an FLT1 with fewer number of injections	• Small • prn treatment regimen
Abedi F[21]	Ranibizumab or bevacizumab*	CFH [rs800292, rs3766404, rs1061170, rs2274700, rs393955], CFHR1-5 [rs10922153], HTRA1 [rs11200638], ARMS2 [rs3793917, 10490924], C3 [rs2230199, rs1047286], C2 [rs547154], CFB [rs641153], F13B [rs6003]	Loss of ≥15 letters of VA	6.4 ± 2.3/1 year#	HTRA1 and ARMS2 risk-allele homozygous associated with worse VA outcome	• Some patients received both bevacizumab and ranibizumab • prn treatment regimen

(Continued)

Table 1. (*Continued*)

Study	Treatment	Genes	Non-responder criteria	Frequency of injections	Results	Limitations
Kloeckener B[23]	Ranibizumab	CFH [rs1061170], HTRA1 [rs11200638], VEGF [1413711], ARMS2 [rs10490924], CFB [rs641153], KDR [rs7671745], FZD4 [rs10898563], LRP5 [rs3736228]	Loss of ≥5 ETDRS letters of VA	4.2 ± 2.3 and 4.1 ± 2.5/1 year (non-responders and responders)#	CFH CC more prevalent among poor responders with worse VA outcomes than in TT and TC; CFH TC and FZD4 GA associated with improved VA	• Not all patients were treatment-naïve • Inconsistent follow-up regimen • No consideration of smoking status • prn treatment regimen
Abedi F[23]	Ranibizumab or bevacizumab*	VEGF-A [rs3024994, rs3025000, rs3025042, rs3025047, rs3025035, rs3025030, rs3025010]	Loss of ≥5 letters of VA	4.3 ± 1/initial 6 months#, 2.4 ± 1.4/ second 6 months	VEGF-A [rs3025000] associated with increased likelihood of <5 letter loss in VA	• Some patients received both bevacizumab and ranibizumab • prn treatment regimen
Wickremasinghe SS[24]	Ranibizumab, bevacizumab or both	APOE [rs429358, rs7412]	—	39 patients with ≤3 and 104 patients with >3/1 year#	ε4 allele associated with increased likelihood of 2-line improvement in VA in early stages of treatment	• Some patients received both bevacizumab and ranibizumab • prn treatment regimen

Smailhodzic D[25]	Ranibizumab	CFH [rs1061170], ARMS2 [rs10490924], VEGF-A [rs699947, rs833069], KDR [rs2071559, rs7671745], LPR5 rs3736228], FZD4 [rs10898563]	—	3/8 weeks#	CFH TT associated with a better VA outcome than CC; CFH and ARMS2 or CFH, ARMS2 and VEGF-A low-risk homozygous with greater improvement in VA than high-risk homozygous; the greater the number of high-risk alleles of CFH and ARMS2, the worse the VA outcomes	• Combined retrospective and prospective study • prn treatment regimen
Zhao L[26]	Ranibizumab or bevacizumab	VEGF-A [rs943080]	No improvement of at least 5 letters or one line on the EDTRS chart at 12 months	Monthly injections for 4 months and then prn based on VA and OCT	Compared with the responder group, the poor-responder group had a higher frequency of the risk (T) allele (Allelic (T) allele $p = 0.019$) and TT	• Retrospective • prn treatment regimen

(Continued)

S. Grob, K. Zhang and S. J. Bakri

Table 1. (*Continued*)

Study	Treatment	Genes	Non-responder criteria	Frequency of injections	Results	Limitations
					genotype ($p = 0.002$ under a recessive model) for the *VEGFA*-rs943080 polymorphism. *VEGFA* expression was 1.8-fold higher in cells with the *VEGFA* rs943080 TT genotype than in cells with the *VEGFA* rs943080 CC genotype ($p = 0.012$).	

*Bevacizumab administered initially in some patients while awaiting insurance approval for ranibizumab.

**No consistent mean number reported.

#Includes 3 initial monthly loading injections.

q4w=every 4 weeks; prn=on as needed basis; VA=visual acuity; OCT=optical coherence tomography.

(rs2230199). Non-responders to treatment were characterized as patients with a decrease of >15 ETDRS letters.[11]

The frequency of the high-risk alleles among participants was higher than in the general population,[28] as all patients enrolled had neovascular AMD. The results of pharmacogenetic analysis did not find statistically significant ($p \leq 0.01$) associations between the SNPs examined and visual acuity (VA) outcomes, anatomic outcomes, or the number of injections. Borderline significance ($p = 0.03$) was found in patients that were homozygous for the risk-alleles of C3 and CFH (although not necessarily simultaneously), for better VA outcomes and for lowest mean change in total foveal thickness, respectively. No statistically significant difference in the number of injections among the different genotypes of the four SNPs was found.[11]

2.1.1 Conclusions

Although the four SNPs examined influence AMD risk, they do not seem to have an impact on response to anti-VEGF therapy, including VA and anatomic outcomes.

2.2. *Pharmacogenetics of complement factor H (Y402H) and treatment of exudative AMD with ranibizumab*

In this retrospective cohort study, treatment-naïve patients with neovascular AMD received intravitreal ranibizumab at initial presentation and prn at follow-up evaluation. Treatment administration, at the discretion of the treating physician, was based on clinical examination and ancillary test results, including: OCT and fluorescein angiography (FA). Patients were followed at unspecified intervals (no bias in frequency of follow-up was found) for a minimum of 9 months with data analysis performed for data collected at initial presentation, 6 months and 9 months. Mouthwash samples were collected for DNA genotypic analysis of buccal cells for CFH (rs1061170).[14]

While there was no statistically significant difference in the post-treatment VA at 6 months or 9 months among the different CFH genotypes, a trend towards increased number of injections required at 9 months and decreased interval between required injections was found among heterozygotes (TC) and homozygotes of the risk-allele (CC).[14]

2.2.1. Conclusions

Although the cohorts at 6 and 9 months were not identical and follow-up of patients was not consistent in this retrospective study, an association between number of intravitreal ranibizumab injections required and the risk allele for CFH was found. No association between genotype and VA outcomes was established.

2.3. *Complement factor H Y402H gene polymorphism and response to intravitreal bevacizumab in exudative AMD*

In this prospective study, patients with treatment-naïve neovascular AMD were treated with intravitreal bevacizumab at 6 week intervals until CNV was inactive. Injections were administered at the discretion of the treating physician. At each follow-up visit, clinical examination and ancillary test results, including OCT and FA, were employed in the determination of treatment necessity. Differences in demographics were found only in that the lowest smoking rate was in the CFH (rs1061170) CC genotype group. Non-responders were characterized as patients that lost ≥3 lines of distance or near VA.[15]

While the proportion of patients that developed CNV in the contralateral eye was highest in the CFH CC genotype group, this was not statistically significant. Statistically significant differences in the percentage of patients that gained three or more lines in distance and near VA and in patients who lost three or more lines were found. Patients in the CFH CC genotype group had worse visual acuity outcomes than the CFH TC and TT genotype groups. In contrast to earlier studies that have reported a higher percentage of classic or predominantly classic lesions in patients with the CFH CC genotype, there was no significant difference in the type of CNV in patients of different genotypes in this study.[15]

2.3.1. Conclusions

Worse visual outcomes are associated with the CFH CC genotype with treatment of neovascular AMD with intravitreal bevacizumab, although a similar association is not observed for the decrease in mean CFT. Additionally, an association between genotype and type of choroidal neovascular lesion was not found.

2.4. *Association of complement factor H and LOC387715 genotypes with response of exudative AMD to intravitreal bevacizumab*

This is a retrospective cohort study of patients with treatment-naïve neovascular AMD treated with intravitreal bevacizumab at 6 week intervals until there was no longer evidence of active neovascularization. Mouthwash samples were collected for genotype analysis for the following two AMD-associated SNPs: (1) CFH (rs1061170) and (2) ARMS2 (rs10490924). Patients were evaluated clinically and fundus photographs and FAs were obtained (no OCT results were reported).[16]

CNV lesions in patients with the lower-risk CFT TT genotype and the higher-risk ARMS2 TT genotype had the largest mean greatest linear dimension (GLD). There was no difference in the percentage of predominantly classic lesions or in the VA at presentation among the different CFH or ARMS2 genotypes. Improvement in mean VA was significantly greater for the CFH TT and TC and ARMS2 GG and GT genotypes than for the homozygous risk-alleles. Mean post-treatment VA for the CFH CC and ARMS2 TT genotypes decreased from pre-treatment VA, however, when adjustment for age, pre-treatment VA and lesion size were made, the difference was not statistically significant for the ARMS2 TT genotype. There was no relationship between the number of risk-alleles and post-treatment VA when CFH and ARMS2 genotypes were combined to determine the total number of risk alleles.[16]

2.4.1. Conclusions

Genetic factors may play a critical role in the efficacy of therapeutic intervention for neovascular AMD, as post-treatment VA was worse in the CFH CC genotype. There were improved visual outcomes in patients with the CFH TT and TC and the ARMS2 GG and GT genotypes. While a lack of association between the CFH genotypes and GLD was reported, an association between the ARMS2 genotypes and GLD were found.

2.5. *Involvement of genetic factors in the response to a variable-dosing ranibizumab treatment regimen for AMD*

This is a 1-year, single-center, genotype-masked, prospective cohort study of patients with subfoveal neovascular AMD treated with intravitreal ranibizumab. Of the 90 participants, 74 were not treatment-naïve, enrolled at ≥3 months after receiving any intravitreal anti-VEGF therapy or ≥6 months after receiving photodynamic therapy (PDT) or intravitreal triamcinolone. Follow-up visits were scheduled monthly, at which time clinical examination, OCT and FA were performed. The decision to inject was based on the criteria applied in the SUSTAIN study: loss of ≥5 ETDRS letters compared to the highest number of letters during the initial 3 months of the study or gain of >100 μm in central subfield retinal thickness (CSRT) compared to the lowest CSRT during the initial 3 months of the study with a pre-requisite for injection for CSRT >225 μm after 3 months of the study. Genotypic analysis, for the CFH (rs1061170) and ARMS2 (rs10490924) SNPs, was performed on dry blood samples.[12]

No significant improvement in VA was observed in the ARMS2 TT genotype. There was statistical significance in the gain in VA in the CFH CC genotype, but this gain was lower than that observed in heterozygous and lower-risk homozygous variants ($p = 0.04$ vs. $p < 0.01$). There was no significant difference in the number of injections administered among the different CFH genotypes.[12]

2.5.1. Conclusions

While patients with the ARMS2 TT genotypes may have decreased CSRT post-treatment with intravitreal ranibizumab, there was no improvement in BCVA, suggesting a possible negative effect secondary to structural changes in the retina, atrophic retinal pigment epithelium (RPE) and/or the loss of photoreceptors. The CFH CC genotype may predispose patients to decreased responsiveness to therapy, necessitating a more aggressive treatment approach.[12]

2.6. Association between high-risk disease loci and response to anti-vascular endothelial growth factor treatment for wet AMD

In this retrospective review of patients with treatment-naïve neovascular AMD, diagnosed by clinical examination and FA, treated with intravitreal injections of ranibizumab and/or bevacizumab, blood samples were collected for genotypic analysis for the following AMD-associated SNPs: CFH (rs1061170), ARMS2 (rs10490924, rs3750848 and del443ins54) and HTRA1 (rs11200638 and rs932275). Intravitreal anti-VEGF injections were given monthly for the first 3 months, then prn based on the stability of the OCT and the absence of subretinal fluid. OCT was performed at initial and follow-up examinations. Non-responders were characterized as patients who lost VA when compared to baseline or those that had a final VA <20/200.[17]

No statistically significant difference in the frequency of the risk-alleles among responders and non-responders was found. Additionally, no significant pharmacogenetic association between the studied SNPs and the efficacy of anti-VEGF therapy was found. Post-injection VA was improved in equal proportions among the CFH CC genotype and the TC and TT genotypes.[17]

2.6.1. Conclusions

The risk-alleles for the CFH, ARMS2, and HTRA1 genes were more prevalent among the patients studied, which is consistent with previous reports, as these genes have been found to be associated with and increased risk of AMD. As no significant pharmacogenetic association was found between the SNPs studied, anti-VEGF therapy for AMD may not need to be guided by genotype.

2.7. *CFH, VEGF and HTRA1 promoter genotype may influence the response to intravitreal ranibizumab for neovascular AMD*

This is a retrospective study in patients with treatment-naïve neovascular AMD patients were treated with intravitreal ranibizumab. A baseline clinical examination, FA, OCT, and indocyanine green angiogram were performed with repeat of clinical examination and OCT at each follow-up visit. Intravitreal ranibizumab was administered monthly for the first 3 months followed by a prn regimen. Determination for necessity of additional injections was prompted by a decrease in VA of ≥5 ETDRS letters and/or persistent or recurrent subretinal fluid, intraretinal cysts or thickening on OCT, or new subretinal hemorrhage on clinical examination. DNA was extracted from peripheral blood lymphocytes and genotype testing for the following SNPs was performed: CFH (rs1061170), VEGF (rs1413711), and HRTA1 (rs11200638). Non-responders were characterized as patients that lost ≥15 ETDRS letters.[13]

While the findings were not statistically significant, a trend towards a more favorable VA outcome (with a larger gain in ETDRS letters) was observed in patients with the high-risk alleles for CFH and VEGF and in heterozygote variants of the HTRA1 polymorphism. No association between the CFH high-risk genotype and number of injections was noted in this study.[13]

2.7.1. Conclusions

High-risk variants of CFH and VEGF may have more favorable VA outcomes, suggesting the possibility of various forms of AMD wherein forms secondary to the aforementioned SNPs, characterized by high levels of VEGF, may respond favorably to anti-VEGF therapy and forms secondary to other genes, not characterized by high levels of VEGF, may respond less favorably.[13]

2.8. *Association of genetic polymorphisms with response to bevacizumab for neovascular AMD in the Chinese population*

A multicenter, prospective study in patients with treatment-naïve neovascular AMD treated with three injections of intravitreal bevacizumab at

6 week intervals. Clinical examination, FA, OCT, and various other ancil-lary testing were performed at the initial and follow-up evaluations. Genotype analysis for the following AMD-associated SNPs was per-formed on peripheral blood samples: CFH (rs800292, rs1061170, rs10801555 and rs1410996), ARMS2 (rs10490924), HTRA1 (rs11200638), VEGF (rs833069 and rs3025039), SERPING1 (rs1005510 and rs2511989) and C3 (rs2230205 and rs2250656).[18]

For the CFH (rs800292) SNP, VA improved for all three genotypes, and was highest for the TT (lower-risk) genotype ($p = 0.009$). Patients with the ARMS2 genotypes TT, TG, and GG (lower-risk) all had signifi-cant improvement in VA with treatment, with the largest mean improve-ment among patients of the TG genotype. Similarly, for the HTRA1 SNP, all genotypes improved with bevacizumab treatment, with the largest improvement found in heterozygotes. Central retinal thickness decreased with treatment among all patients, although no association between the different genotypes of the tested SNPs was found. No asso-ciation between treatment outcomes and the VEGF, SERPING1, and C3 SNPs was found.[18]

2.8.1. Conclusion

An association between the studied SNPs and response to treatment of AMD with intravitreal bevacizumab exists and for the ARMS2 and HTRA1 SNPs, heterozygotes had the greatest improvement. This finding may support the belief of "heterozygote advantage." SNPs may alter the expression of certain proteins, possibly influencing treatment outcome.[18]

2.9. VEGF-A polymorphisms predict short-term functional response to intravitreal ranibizumab in exudative AMD

In this prospective, single-center study of patients with treatment-naïve neovascular AMD, patients received three intravitreal loading doses of ranibizumab at monthly intervals. OCT was utilized in diagnosis of neo-vascular AMD and was performed at 28 ± 2 days from each injection. Peripheral blood samples were obtained and testing for two VEGF-A (rs699947 and rs1570360) SNPs was performed.[19]

A statistically significant association between the rs699947 SNP and VA outcome was established, as patients with the heterozygous and non-wild-type homozygous genotypes had better responses to treatment than the wild-type genotype.[19]

2.9.1. Conclusion

The presence of a particular VEGF-A genotype may result in a more favorable response to intravitreal anti-VEGF therapy, supporting the theory that response to anti-VEGF treatment of AMD may be dependent on genotype, and personalized therapy can be implemented in an attempt to improve visual outcomes.

2.10. *The influence of genetics on response to treatment with ranibizumab (Lucentis) for AMD: the Lucentis genotype study*

In this two-site, prospective observational study of patients with treatment-naïve neovascular AMD, patients were treated with intravitreal ranibizumab. Intravitreal ranibizumab was administered at the time of initial screening and 1-month later, followed by prn treatment at monthly follow-up examinations as determined by the following criteria: presence of intraretinal fluid, subretinal fluid, or retinal thickening on OCT; presence of new subretinal hemorrhage; active, new subretinal CNV membrane documented on FA and a loss of ≥5 ETDRS letters of VA compared to prior visit. OCT was performed at the screening, 1-month examination, and on a monthly basis at follow-up examinations. DNA genotype analysis was performed on peripheral blood samples. A very large number of SNPs were tested, with the following as the major genes: CFH (rs1065489, rs3753394 and rs3766404), ARMS2 (rs10490924), C3 (rs1389623 and rs2230205), VEGF-A (rs3025033, rs833069 and rs833068), CTGF (connective tissue growth factor) (rs9399005), FLT1 (VEGF receptor-1) (rs9319428, rs9319425, rs622227, rs2387632, rs10507386, rs615529 and rs7995976), THBS1 (thombospondin-1) (rs1478604), and FGFR2 (fibroblast growth factor receptor-2) (rs1047100 and rs2912762). CFH, ARMS2, and C3 are characterized as AMD susceptibility genes while VEGF-A, CTGH, FLT1, THBS1, and FGFR2 are characterized as angiogenesis genes.[20]

The minor allele for the CFH (rs1065489) and CTGF genes appeared to confer a worse visual outcome. For the C3 (rs2230205) SNP, patients with the minor allele appeared to have a greater reduction in retinal thickness at 6 and 12 months. Patients with the minor alleles of VEGF-A and FLT1 required fewer intravitreal injections (over 12 months) while patients with the minor allele of the CFH gene required more injections. Several SNPs of FLT1 are associated with persistent leakage on FA.[20]

2.10.1. Conclusion

The CFH risk-allele is implicated in conferring a poorer visual outcome, as also seen with a SNP in the CTGF gene. The minor allele of C3 is associated with reduced retinal thickening. Certain FLT1 SNPs are associated with poorer visual outcome. VEGF-A, FLT1, and CFH could possibly be utilized to predict which eyes will require fewer injections and thus time between follow-up visits can be increased.

2.11. *Genetic influences on the outcome of anti-vascular endothelial growth factor treatment in neovascular AMD*

This is a 1-year prospective cohort study of patients with treatment-naïve neovascular AMD that were treated with three initial monthly intravitreal injections of ranibizumab or bevacizumab (21% of patients received bevacizumab initially while awaiting insurance approval for ranibizumab) and prn treatment for the remainder of the study. Re-treatment criteria include: loss of ≥5 ETDRS letters of VA, persistent or recurrent intraretinal or subretinal fluid on OCT, or the presence of new or persistent hemorrhage on examination. Follow-up examinations were scheduled at 1-month intervals with a 2-week extension if patients were stable and did not require re-treatment. Many different SNPs, including CFH (rs800292, rs3766404, rs1061170, rs2274700 and rs393955), CFHR1-5 (rs10922153), HTRA1 (rs11200638), ARMS2 (rs3793917 and 10490924), C3 (rs2230199 and rs1047286), C2 (rs547154), CFB (rs641153), and F13B (rs6003) were studied. Non-responders were defined as patients that lost ≥15 letters of VA.[21]

The HTRA1 and ARMS2 SNPs were the only SNPs that demonstrated a statistically significant relationship with visual outcome at 1 year, patients homozygous for the risk-allele had worse visual outcomes.[21]

2.11.1. Conclusion

Patients with neovascular AMD who are homozygous for the risk-alleles of the HTRA1 and ARMS2 SNPs are more likely to have worse visual outcomes with intravitreal ranibizumab treatment.

2.12. *Genetic association with response to intravitreal ranibizumab in patients with neovascular AMD*

This is a prospective study of patients with neovascular AMD treated with intravitreal ranibizumab. Most patients were treatment-naïve (13.6% eyes had received previous treatment with non-ranibizumab therapies). Patients received treatment at initial examination and at follow-up visits prn. While follow-up visits were scheduled monthly, there was some variation secondary to patient needs. Treatment was administered when signs of active lesions were evident, this includes subretinal fluid, cystoid macular edema, sub- or intraretinal bleeding or active lesion on FA. OCT was performed at baseline and at follow-up examinations. Poor responders were defined as patients that lost ≥5 ETDRS letters of vision. Genotype analysis was performed on DNA obtained from venous blood samples. The following genes were evaluated: CFH (rs1061170), HTRA1 (rs11200638), VEGF (rs1413711), ARMS2 (rs10490924), CFB (rs641153), KDR (kinase insert domain receptor; VEGFR2 precursor) (rs7671745), FZD4 (frizzled homolog 4) (rs10898563), and LRP5 (low-density lipoprotein receptor-related protein 5) (rs3736228). The latter three genes are known to play a role in angiogenesis and vascularization.[22]

The prevalence of the risk-allele among the patients with neovascular AMD was greater than the controls for CFH, HTRA1, ARMS2, LRP5, and CFB. The increased prevalence of the CFH CC genotype among the poor responders was statistically significant. There was a statistically significant difference in visual outcomes in the CFH genotypes, with patients who were CFH CC with worse visual outcomes than CFH TC and TT genotypes. Patients that were heterozygous for both of the SNPs in CFH and FZD4 (TC/GA) were more likely to have improved VA. No difference in the injection frequency among poor responders and good responders was found.[22]

2.12.1. Conclusion

The CFH CC genotype is associated with a poorer visual outcome and the heterozygous genotype of the CFH and FZD4 SNPs is associated with a more favorable visual outcome.

2.13. *Variants in the VEGF-A gene and treatment outcome after anti-VEGF treatment for neovascular AMD*

In this single-center, prospective cohort study, patients with neovascular AMD were treated with either intravitreal ranibizumab or bevacizumab (19.4% of patients received bevacizumab initially while awaiting insurance approval for ranibizumab). Intravitreal anti-VEGF therapy was given monthly for the first 3 months followed by prn dosing. Criteria for re-treatment included: loss of >5 letters of vision, increased central retinal thickness of >100 μm, the presence of retinal fluid on OCT or new or persistent hemorrhage on examination. Follow-up examinations were scheduled at 1-month intervals with a 2-week extension if patients were stable and did not require re-treatment. Clinical examination and OCT was performed at baseline and all follow-up examinations. Seven SNPs in the VEGF-A gene (rs3024994, rs3025000, rs3025042, rs3025047, rs3025035, rs3025030 and rs3025010) were selected for evaluation. Non-responders were defined as patients with loss of ≥5 letters of vision.[23]

At 6 months, only the rs3025000 SNP was found to have a statistically significant ($p < 0.007$) association with visual outcomes. This SNP was also the only one associated with an increased likelihood of patients belonging to the responder [vs. non-responder] sub-category at 3, 6, and 12 months. The number of intravitreal injections administered did not differ among the TT or TC and CC genotypes of the rs3025000 SNP. The patients of the TT or TC genotypes at rs3025000 SNP of VEGF-A had similar outcomes of the similarly matched patients in the ANCHOR and MARINA studies and better outcomes than patients of the CC genotype.[23]

2.13.1. Conclusion

A potential pharmacogenetic relationship between the rs3025000 SNP of VEGF-A and visual outcome after treatment with intravitreal ranibizumab (and bevacizumab) in patients with neovascular AMD exists.

2.14. *Common variant in VEGFA and response to anti-VEFF therapy for neovascular AMD*

In this retrospective study of 223 patients with neovascular AMD, visual outcomes and central foveal thickness were evaluated in association with the genotype of the *VEGFA* gene and treatment response.[26] Patients were treated with monthly injections of anti-VEGF therapy with either ranibizumab or bevacizumab for a total of 4 months. Thereafter, the patients received injections as needed if their vision dropped at least five letters on the ETDRS chart or intraretinal or subretinal fluid was present on optical coherence tomography (OCT). Responders were defined as patients who had an improvement in best corrected visual acuity (BCVA) of at least five letters or one line on the EDTRS visual acuity chart along with resolution of intraretinal or subretinal fluid over 12 months. Patients who did not meet the definition of responders were classified as poor-responders. The vision of responders (n = 148) improved while the vision of poor-responders (n = 75) worsened (p <0.001). Responders on average had a decrease in central foveal thickness (CFT), while poor-responders had an increase in CFT (p <0.001). Compared with the responder group, the poor-responder group had a higher frequency of the risk (T) allele (Allelic p = 0.019) and TT genotype (P = 0.002 under a recessive model) for the *VEGFA*-rs943080 polymorphism. *VEGFA* expression was 1.8-fold higher in cells with the *VEGFA* rs943080 TT genotype than in cells with the *VEGFA* rs943080 CC genotype (p = 0.012). Age, gender, smoking, diabetes mellitus, and hypertension did not play a significant role in treatment response, but BMI was found to be significantly different between responders and poor-responders (p = 0.033).[26]

2.14.1. Conclusion

A potential pharmacogenetic relationship between the rs943080 SNP of VEGF-A and visual outcome after treatment with intravitreal ranibizumab or bevacizumab in patients with neovascular AMD is demonstrated.[26]

2.15. *Variants in the APOE gene are associated with improved outcome after anti-VEGF treatment for neovascular AMD*

In this prospective study of patients with subfoveal neovascular AMD, visual outcomes and association with SNPs of the APOE gene (rs429358 and rs7412) were examined. Patients were treated with intravitreal ranibizumab, bevacizumab, or both (at different times). Intravitreal anti-VEGF therapy was administered monthly for the first 3 months in 75% of patients followed by prn treatment. As no difference in the frequency of the APOE alleles was observed among the group of patients that received only ranibizumab as compared to the patients who received both ranibizumab and bevacizumab, the patients were combined and analyzed as a single cohort (No OCT results were reported).[24]

A statistically significant difference in visual outcome, with a greater proportion of patients with a two-line improvement in visual outcome with at least one copy of the ε4 allele than in patients with at least one copy of the ε2 allele, was observed. The presence of the ε4 allele was significantly associated with a greater likelihood of improvement in vision at 3 months, but not at 6 or 12 months. For patients in whom both eyes were treated and evaluated, only the eye with the worse visual outcome was included in the study.[24]

2.15.1. Conclusion

The APOE genotype is significantly associated with visual outcome in patients with neovascular AMD. The ε4 allele is confers an increased likelihood of a two-line improvement in VA in early stages of treatment.

2.16. *Cumulative effect of risk alleles in CFH, ARMS2, and VEGF-A on the response to ranibizumab treatment in AMD*

This is a combination retrospective and prospective case series study in treatment-naïve patients with neovascular AMD that were treated with intravitreal ranibizumab monthly for the first 3 months followed by prn treatment for active CNV as observed on clinical examination, OCT, or FA. DNA analysis was performed on venous blood samples for the following AMD-associated SNPs: CFH (rs1061170), ARMS2 (rs10490924), VEGF-A (rs699947 and rs833069), KDR (kinase insert domain-containing receptor/fetal liver kinas, VEGFR-2) (rs2071559 and rs7671745), LPR5 (involved with angiogenesis) (rs3736228), and FZD4 (rs10898563).[25]

Increased age was associated with significant loss in VA after three monthly ranibizumab injections. Heterozygous variants of the ARMS2 (GT) and KDR (GA) genotypes were older at the time of initial treatment than homozygous high-risk variants. Individuals carrying the CFH low-risk allele (TT) had a better visual outcome than those carrying the high-risk allele (CC). Additionally, patients that were low-risk homozygous for CFH and ARMS2 or CFH, ARMS2 and VEGF-A had significantly more improvement in VA than high-risk homozygote counterparts. Statistical significance between the total number of high-risk alleles of CFH and ARMS2 and age at treatment initiation was found. No significant associations between visual outcome and the LRP5 and FZD4 SNPs were found.[25]

2.16.1. Conclusion

A significant pharmacogenetic relationship between carriers of the high-risk alleles of CFH, ARMS2, and VEGF-A and poorer response to intra-vitreal anti-VEGF treatment with ranibizumab exists, with this effect being additive. Additionally, patients with high-risk alleles for these SNPs meet criteria for treatment of neovascular AMD at a younger age.

3. Discussion

In recent years, several AMD-associated genes have been identified. Specific SNPs in these genes are more prevalent among patients with

AMD and have been found to confer a predisposition to the development of AMD. Of the studied SNPs, the strongest associations have been found for the following genes: CFH, C3, ARMS2, and HTRA1.[8,31–37] The recognition of genetic variations among patients with AMD has led to the search for a pharmacogenetic relationship between response to AMD therapies and genotype.

While the exact pathophysiologic mechanisms for the pharmacogenetic relationships between specific SNPs and response to anti-VEGF therapy are unknown, theories describing this effect have been postulated. Lee AY[14] hypothesized that the increased inflammation may be found in patients with complement-related AMD-risk alleles favoring recurrence of neovascularization secondary to increased VEGF levels,[14] thus diminishing the response to anti-VEGF therapy in these patients. Additional hypotheses concerning the influence of the ARMS2 genotype on response to anti-VEGF therapy embrace the necessity of the ARMS2 protein in the prevention of damage. The ARMS2 protein is localized to the outer membrane of mitochondria and as a decrease in mitochondrial number and size has been reported in the retinas of patients with AMD,[28] it has been hypothesized that the mechanism of effect of the ARMS2 SNP on response to anti-VEGF treatment may result from oxidative damage to photoreceptors and the RPE.[21,27]

Interest in the investigation of the pharmacogenetics of the response to intravitreal anti-VEGF treatment developed, in part, after studies found variations in intravitreal VEGF levels in patients with AMD and matched controls without AMD.[44,45] It has been postulated that these variations may explain the requirement of a greater number of injections to achieve treatment response in some patients. Some studies have found a significant relationship between the number of injections necessary to achieve treatment response and genotype[14,20] while other studies have found no relationship.[11,12,15,16,21,23] While it is possible that additional or more frequent intravitreal anti-VEGF injections might be necessary to achieve improvement in VA, there is also the possibility that more aggressive treatment is not beneficial.[16] This brings to light the criteria used to determine treatment response and/or adequate response, or lack thereof, as it influences further management.

With the intent of quantifying response to anti-VEGF therapy, some studies identify patients as non-responders/poor responders. The definition of a non-responder varies across studies with some defining these patients as those that simply have worsening of VA from baseline[11] or no improvement in VA[16,17] to those that lose ≥5–15 letters of VA.[13,15,21–23] Variations in criteria that define non-responders may complicate result interpretation. For example, in the Nischler C[15] study, non-responders were defined as patients that lost ≥3 lines of VA and in the Brantley MA[16] study, non-responders were defined as patients that did not have improvement in VA. Nischler C[15] reported that 41% of patients that were homozygous for the risk-allele of CFH and 28% that were homozygous for the low-risk allele of CFH were non-responders whereas Brantley MA[16] reported that 89.5% of patients that were homozygous for the risk-allele of CFH and 50% that were homozygous for the low-risk allele for CFH were non-responders. Accurately identifying patients who are not responsive to intravitreal anti-VEGF therapy is important for optimizing outcome as alternative therapies or treatment regimens may need to be implemented.

It is evident that the study design has a significant impact on the applicability of results and it is an important consideration when deciding to implement changes to improve patient care. Small, retrospective studies with short follow-up and lack of standardization or control for confounding factors can limit the utility of study results.

In all of the studies discussed, current standard doses of medication were used, intravitreal ranibizumab dosing was 0.5 mg/0.05 ml and bevacizumab dosing was 1.25 mg/0.05 ml. Unfortunately, the results of these studies may not be applicable to all patients as, in all but four of these studies, a prn treatment regimen was implemented. Previous investigations have consistently shown a trend towards better visual and anatomic outcomes in patients on a standardized treatment regimen (monthly/q4w) compared to a prn regimen.[5,39,40] Therefore, additional studies should aim to prospectively evaluate the response to a standardized treatment regimen, in an attempt to better delineate the pharmacogenetics of AMD treatment.

A prospective study design is ideal and should be performed whenever possible. Of the studies discussed, six were retrospective in nature,[13,14,16,17,25,26] although one had a small population of patients examined prospectively. Limitations of a retrospective study include decreased ability to establish cause and effect, control exposure, and control bias. In a retrospective study, it is difficult to assess a temporal relationship. Retrospective studies are not designed to examine the cause-effect relationship; therefore while correlations can be made, determination of cause and effect is problematic. It is also difficult to control exposure and outcome assessment in retrospective studies, and investigators must rely on the availability and accuracy of the medical record. Data calculation and interpretation becomes problematic in retrospective studies due to lack of bias control and confounding factors, as there is often no pre-specified standardization of procedure, randomization, or blinding.

Standardization of procedure is important for data analysis as a lack of such complicates categorization and outcome. Inconsistencies in medication used are notable in three studies.[21,23,24] A proportion of patients in these studies were treated with both intravitreal bevacizumab and ranibizumab at different times throughout the study. Some studies have demonstrated comparable outcomes of treatment with intravitreal ranibizumab and bevacizumab,[5,40] but to improve study design, exclusion of patients receiving both treatments may be ideal. Similarly, in two studies, patients were not treatment-naïve.[12,22] Patients in these studies, had previously received treatment for neovascular AMD with intravitreal anti-VEGF injections (including pegaptanib), intravitreal steroids and/or PDT. This likely complicates the results as previous studies have demonstrated that patients may show a greater response during the initial treatment phase.

In consideration of earlier reports that sharp changes in VA and central retinal thickness occur after only three monthly injections,[5] some of the studies only evaluated patients after three monthly injections.[18,19,25] As most patients with neovascular AMD receive treatment over extended periods of time, the data from these studies may not be practical for use in developing a personalized treatment plan. The potential for insignificant differences in the response to anti-VEGF treatment among different genotypes, when examined over an extended period of time, exists. Therefore, these studies limit the applicability of the results in many patients with neovascular AMD.

The applicability of the data obtained in the above studies is also limited by demographic differences. Many of the genetic studies that led to the identification of AMD-associated SNPs were performed in Caucasians. As a majority of the studies exploring the pharmacogenetics of response to anti-VEGF therapy, except Tian J,[18] studied a mostly Caucasian population, the results may not be applicable to patients of all races.

Another consideration in an attempt to limit confounding factors is the categorization of patients by certain risk factors. For example, five studies did not consider smoking status of participants.[12,16,17,19,22] Earlier studies report that previous or current smoking impacts the course of AMD.[41,42] Not controlling this factor may explain the inability to find a pharmacogenetic relationship between genotype and response to anti-VEGF therapy or the presence of only a weak pharmacogenetic relationship.

Of the studies in pharmacogenetics of anti-VEGF treatment of neovascular AMD discussed above, none had a placebo-controlled group and most were observational studies of patients on a prn treatment regimen. Due to these limitations, the ability to consistently and accurately detect a significant pharmacogenetic relationship is diminished. A large, prospective, double-blind, placebo-controlled, interventional study with extended follow-up, in patients with neovascular AMD may provide the power necessary to detect a significant association between genotype and response to anti-VEGF therapy. In addition, further genetic analyses, simultaneously involving multiple genes, may demonstrate an additive or antagonistic effect. Stratification based on lifestyle factors, such as smoking status, and antioxidant intake should be performed to more accurately analyze data. It may also be beneficial to group patients according to stage of disease and size of lesions. Genome-wide study analysis in non-Caucasian populations may lead to the identification of neovascular AMD-associated SNPs and their prevalence in these populations, improving the validity of study results and its relevance to non-Caucasian populations. Additionally, variables such as presenting VA and patient age may also contribute to visual outcome, complicating the pharmacogenetic relationship between certain SNPs and treatment response to anti-VEGF therapy.[24] The combination of the data collected from these additional GWAS and further investigation of VEGF-A gene expression is crucial for better understanding of the pharmacogenetics of treatment response in neovascular AMD.

Variability in results reported in different studies complicates the decision to personalize therapy for neovascular AMD. The main genes investigated have been implicated in increasing the risk of AMD, but their involvement in the biologic pathways contributing to the development of AMD may be inconsequential. For this reason, it is important to continue investigating the pharmacogenetics of AMD and to identify gene products more directly involved in the biologic pathways of neovascular AMD.

As new data emerges and it becomes evident that genetic background may in fact influence an individual's response to treatment, personalized therapy offers the potential for significantly improved treatment outcome. Early identification of non-responders/poor responders is essential for the implementation of personalized therapy, in hopes of maximizing visual outcome and minimizing number of treatments and risks associated with them. Reduction of treatment burden and cost can be optimized through personalized therapy, as the possibility of eliminating the loading phase of therapy exists for patients that demonstrate a significant early response to therapy.

4. References

1. Veritti, D., Sarao, V., Lanzetta, P. Neovascular age-related macular degeneration. *Ophthalmologica* **227**(suppl 1), 11–20 (2012).
2. Zarbin, M.A. Current concepts in the pathogenesis of age-related macular degeneration. *Arch Ophthalmol* **122**, 598–614 (2004).
3. Grisanti, S., Tatar, O. The role of vascular endothelial growth factor and other endogenous interplayers in age-related macular degeneration. *Prog Retin Eye Res* **27**, 327–390 (2008).
4. Saeed, M.U., Gkaragkani, E., Ali, K. Emerging roles for antiangiogenesis factors in management of ocular disease. *Clinical Ophthalmology* **7**, 533–543 (2013).
5. CATT Research Group, Martin, D.F., Maguire, M.G., Fine, S.L. Ranibizumab and bevacizumab for neovascular age-related macular degeneration. *N Engl J Med* **364**(20), 1897–1908 (2011).
6. Lazzeri, S., Nardi, M., Bocci, G. Pharmacogenetic labyrinth of neovascular age-related macular degeneration therapy: how to escape and move forward? *Pharmacogenomics* **14**(11), 1239–1242 (2013).
7. Lux, A., Llacer, H., Leussen, F., *et al.* Non-responders to bevacizumab (Avastin) therapy of choroidal neovascular lesions. *Br J Ophthalmol* **91**(10), 1318–1322 (2007).

8. Deangelis, M.M., Silveira, A.C., Carr, E.A., Kim, I.K. Genetics of age-related macular degeneration: current concepts, future directions. *Semin Ophthalmol* **26**, 77–93 (2011).

9. Haddad, S., Checn, C.A., Santangelo, S.L., Seddon, J.M. The genetics of age-related macular: a review of progress to date. *Surv Ophthalmol* **51**, 316–363 (2006).

10. Swaroop, A., Chew, E.Y., Rickman, C.B., Abecasis, G.R. Unraveling a multifactorial late-onset disease: from genetic susceptibility to disease mechanisms for age-related macular degeneration. *Annu Rev Genomics Hum Genet* **10**, 19–43 (2009).

11. Hagstrom, S.A., Ying, G., Pauer, G.J., *et al.* Pharmacogenetics for genes associated with age-related macular degeneration in the comparison of AMD treatments trials (CATT). *Ophthalmology* **120**(3), 593–599 (2013).

12. Teper, S.J., Nowinska, A., Pilat, J., *et al.* Involvement of genetic factors in the response to a variable-dosing ranibizumab treatment regimen for age-related macular degeneration. *Mol Vis* **16**, 2598–2604 (2010).

13. McKibbin, M., Ali, M., Bansal, S., *et al.* CFH, VEGF and HTRA1 promoter genotype may influence the response to intravitreal ranibizumab therapy for neovascular age-related macular degeneration. *Br J Ophthalmol* **96**, 208–212 (2012).

14 Lee, A.Y., Raya, A.K., Kymes, S.M., *et al.* Pharmacogenetics of complement factor H (Y402H) and treatment of exudative age-related macular degeneration with ranibizumab. *Br J Ophthalmol* **93**, 610–613 (2009).

15 Nischler, C., Oberkofler, H., Ortner, C., *et al.* Complement factor H Y402H gene polymorphism and response to intravitreal bevacizumab in exudative age-related macular degeneration. *Acta Ophthalmol* **89**, e344–349 (2011).

16. Brantley, M.A., Fang, A.M.M., King, J.M., *et al.* Association of complement factor H and LOC387715 genotypes with response of exudative age-related macular degeneration to intravitreal bevacizumab. *Ophthalmology* **114**, 2168–2173 (2007).

17. Orlin, A., Hadley, D., Chang, W., *et al.* Association between high-risk disease loci and response to anti-vascular endothelial growth factor treatment for wet age-related macular degeneration. *Retina* **32**, 4–9 (2012).

18. Tian, J., Qin, X., Fang, K., *et al.* Association of genetic polymorphisms with response to bevacizumab for neovascular age-related macular degeneration in the Chinese population. *Pharmacogenomics* **13**(7), 779–787 (2012).

19. Lazzeri, A., Figus, M., Orlandi, P., *et al.* VEGF-A polymorphisms predict short-term functional response to intravitreal ranibizumab in exudative age-related macular degeneration. *Pharmacogenomics* **14**(6), 623–630 (2013).

20. Francis, P.J. The influence of genetics on response to treatment with ranibizumab (Lucentis) for age-related macular degeneration: the Lucentis genotype study (an American Ophthalmological Society thesis). *Trans Am Ophthalmol Soc* **109**, 115–156 (2011).
21. Abedi, F., Wickremasinghe, S., Richardson, A.J., *et al*. Genetic influences on the outcome of anti-vascular endothelial growth factor treatment in neovascular age-related macular degeneration. *Ophthalmology* **120**, 1641–1648 (2013).
22. Kloeckener-Gruissem, B., Barthelmes, D., Labs, S., *et al*. Genetic association with response to intravitreal ranibizumab in patients with neovascular AMD. *IOVS* **52**(7), 4694–4702 (2011).
23. Abedi, F., Wickremasinghe, S.S., Richardson, A.J., *et al*. Variants in the VEGF-A gene and treatment for neovascular age-related macular degeneration. *Ophthalmology* **120**, 115–121 (2013).
24. Wickremaskinghe, S.S., Xie, J., Lim, J., *et al*. Variants in the APOE gene are associated with improved outcome after anti-VEGF treatment for neovascular AMD. *IOVS* **52**(7), 4072–4079 (2011).
25. Smailhodzic, D., Muether, P.S., Chen, J., *et al*. Cumulative effect of risk alleles in CFH, ARMS2, and VEGF-A on the response to ranibizumab treatment in age-related macular degeneration. *Ophthalmology* **119**, 2304–2311 (2012).
26. Zhao, L., Grob, S., Avery, R., *et al*. Common variant in VEGFA and response to anti-VEGF therapy for neovascular age-related macular degeneration. *Curr Mol Med* **13**, 929–934 (2013).
27. Tong, Y., Liao, J., Zhang, Y., *et al*. LOC387715/HTRA1 gene polymorphisms and susceptibility to age-related macular degeneration: a HuGE review and meta-analysis. *Mol Vis* [serial online] 2010;**16**:1958-81. Available at: http://www. Molvis.org/molvis/v16/a213/. Accessed August 24, 2013.
28. Feher, J., Kovacs, I., Artico, M., *et al*. Mitochondrial alterations of retinal pigment epithelium in age-related macular degeneration. *Neurobiol Aging* **27**, 983–993 (2006).
29. Gu, J., Pauer, G.J., Yue, X., *et al*. Clinical Genomic and Proteomic AMD Study Group. Assessing susceptibility to age-relate macular degeneration with proteomic and genomic biomarkers. *Mol Cell Proteomics* **8**, 1338–1349 (2009).
30. Awh, C.C., Lane, A., Hawken, S., *et al*. CFH an ARMS2 genetic polymorphisms predict response to antioxidants and zinc in patients with age-related macular degeneration. *Ophthalmology* (2013). pii: S0161-6420(13)00679-9. doi: 10.1016/j.ophtha.2013.07.039 [epub ahead of print].

94   *S. Grob, K. Zhang and S. J. Bakri*

31. Baird, P.N., Hageman, G.S., Franzco, R.H.G. New era for personalized medicine: the diagnosis and management of age-related macular degeneration. *Clin Exp Ophthalmol* **37**(8), 814–821 (2009).
32. Gold, B., Merriam, J.E., Zernant, J., *et al.* Variation in factor B (BF) and complement component 2 (C2) genes is associated with age-related macular degeneration. *Nat Genet* **38**, 458–462 (2006).
33. Haines, J.L., Hauser, M.A., Schmidt, S., *et al.* Complement factor H variant increases the risk of age-related macular degeneration. *Science* **308**, 419–421 (2005).
34. Yang, Z., Camp, N.J., Sun, H., *et al.* A variant of the HTRA1 gene increases susceptibility to age-related macular degeneration. *Science* **314**, 992–993 (2006).
35. Despriet, D.D., Klaver, C.C., Witteman, J.C., *et al.* Complement factor H polymorphism, complement activators, and risk of age-related macular degeneration. *JAMA* **296**, 301–309 (2006).
36. Ding, X., Patel, M., Chan, C.C. Molecular pathology of age-related macular degeneration. *Prog Retin Eye Res* **28**, 1–18 (2009).
37. Schwartz, S.G., Brantley, M.A. Jr. Pharmacogenetics and age-related macular degeneration. *J Ophthalmol* (2011); 2011: 252549. doi: 10. 1155/2011/252549. Epub 2011 Oct 20.
38. Martin, D.F., Maguire, M.G., Ying, G.S., *et al.* Ranibizumab and bevacizumab for neovascular age-related macular degeneration. *N Engl J Med* **364**, 1897–1908 (2011).
39. Martin, D.F., Maguire, M.G., Fine, S.L., *et al.* Ranibizumab and bevacizumab for treatment of neovascular age-related macular degeneration: two-year results. *Ophthalmology* **119**, 1388–1398 (2012).
40. Chakravarthy, U., Harding, S.P., Rogers, C.A., *et al.* Ranibizumab versus bevacizumab to treat neovascular age-related macular degeneration: one-year findings from the IVAN randomized trial. *Ophthalmology* **119**, 1399–1411 (2012).
41. Chakravarthy, U., Harding, S.P., Rogers, C.A., *et al.* Alternative treatments to inhibit VEGF in age-related choroidal neovascularization: 2-year findings of the IVAN randomized trial. *Lancet* (2013) pii: S0140-6736(13)61501-9. doi: 10.1016/S0140-6736(13)61501-9. [Epub ahead of print].
42. Chakravarthy, U., Wong, T.Y., Fletcher, A., *et al.* Clinical risk factors for age-related macular degeneration: a systematic review and metaanalysis. *BMC Ophthalmol* **10**, 31 (2010).
43. Clemons, T.E., Milton, R.C., Klein, R., *et al.* Risk factors for the incidence of advanced age-related macular degeneration in the Age-Related Eye

Disease Study (AREDS) AREDS report no. 19. *Ophthalmology* **112**, 533–539 (2005).

44. Funk, M., Karl, D., Georgopoulos, M., *et al.* Neovascular age-related macular degeneration: intraocular cytokines and growth factors and the influence of therapy with ranibizumab. *Ophthalmology* **116**, 2393–2399 (2009).

45. Tong, J.P., Chan, W.M., Liu, D.T., *et al.* Aqueous humor levels of vascular endothelial growth factor and pigment epithelium-derived factor in polypoidal choroidal vasculopathy and choroidal neovascularization. *Am J Ophthalmol* **141**, 456–462 (2006).

Chapter 4: Dry Eye Therapy

Seanna Grob, * *Igor Kozak*[†] *and Kang Zhang*[‡]

Massachusetts Eye and Ear Infirmary,
Harvard Medical School, Boston, MA
[†]*King Khaled Eye Specialist Hospital,*
Riyadh, Saudi Arabia
[‡]*Shiley Eye Institute, University of California San Diego,*
La Jolla, CA

1. Introduction

Dry eye disease (DED) is one of the most common clinical indications for ophthalmic consultations. The prevalence of DED has been reported in the range of 4–30% in different populations, with a prevalence of 27.5% in an Indonesian population, 21.6% in females and 12.5% in males in a Japanese population, and 4.3%, 10%, and 7.8% in separate male, veteran and female populations in the United States respectively.[1-3] [4,5] Studies have also shown an increase of the prevalence of DED with age.[5,6] The Women's Health Study[6] and the Physicians Health Study[7] are some of the larger epidemiological studies of DED which have estimated that approximately 3.23 million females and 1.68 million males ≥50 years old suffer from DED in the United States. Millions more are impacted with less severe symptoms or have an episodic manifestation of the disease that is only symptomatic with environmental or other stressors, such as low humidity.

Dry eye symptoms are often described by patients as affecting their ability to read, drive at night, and work with computers. Patients with DED express feelings of frustration, unhappiness, depression, decrease in confidence and difficulty dealing with chronic pain.[8] DED thus has a considerable impact on visual function, daily activities, productivity in the workplace, physical and social functioning, and quality of life (QOL).

Studies on QOL have shown that severe DED impacts a patient in a similar way to that of hospital dialysis and moderate to severe angina.[9,10] Moderate and moderate to severe angina, or chest pain, have a cormorbid-ity-adjusted utility score of 0.75 and 0.72 and DED utility scores range from 0.78 for mild DED to 0.62 for severe DED.[10]

In addition, the cost of DED is considerable. The overall annual burden of managing DED in the United States has been estimated at 55.4 billion dollars, which includes doctors visits, medications, office or surgical procedures, and costs for loss of productivity.[11] There are additional costs that are difficult to evaluate, such as the cost of pain medications for this condition. Also, there is currently only one FDA-approved medication, Restasis®, for the treatment of DED and this was approved over a decade ago in 2002. Therefore, there currently is an unmet need for developing new and more effective treatments for DED. New therapies could significantly reduce drug costs, medical care costs, and improve patients' productivity and quality of life.

2. Background of DED

2.1. *Definition of DED*

The International Dry Eye Workshop (DEWS) of 2007 defined DED as "a multifactorial disease of the tears and ocular surface that results in symptoms of discomfort, visual disturbance, and tear film instability with potential damage to the ocular surface. It is accompanied by increased osmolarity of the tear film and inflammation of the ocular surface."[12] DED is recognized as a disturbance of the lacrimal functional unit (LFU), which is "an integrated system comprising the lacrimal glands, ocular surface (cornea and conjunctiva), eyelids and blink mechanism that spreads the tears, meibomian glands, and the motor and sensory nerves that innervate them."[13] A functioning LFU preserves the integrity of the tear film, the clarity and contour of the cornea, and the quality of the image projected onto the retina.[13–15] When this unit is disturbed, patients experience dry eye or foreign body sensation, burning, stinging, itching, pain or ocular soreness, intolerance to contact lenses, blurred vision and photophobia, with more serious complications including corneal erosions, corneal ulcers, corneal scarring, and decrease in visual acuity.

2.2. Types of DED

The tear film provides several benefits to the ocular surface. It functions as a protective layer that washes away irritants and pathogens, dilutes toxins and allergens, and regulates the normal ocular flora. It is also an important refractive interface that is responsible for maintaining a smooth optical surface. However, our understanding of the complex factors involved in the normal functioning of the tear film is still evolving.

Previously, the tear film was described as a tri-layered structure, including the outer lipid layer, the intermediate aqueous layer, and the inner mucin layer, each with a unique and important function. More recent research has proposed the tear film as a uniform gel, which is secreted by conjunctival goblet cells and is mixed with fluids and proteins secreted by the lacrimal, meibomian, and accessory glands. This mixture of secretory products lubricates (mucins), heals (epidermal growth factor [EGF]), and protects the ocular surface from infection (lactoferrin, defensins, Immunoglobulin A) and excessive inflammation (interleukin-1 receptor [IL-1RA], transforming growth factor-β [TGF-β], and tissue inhibitor of matrix metalloproteinase 1 [TIMP-1]).[16]

Not only does the complex mixture of the tear film have to be present, but the entire LFU needs to be intact as well. An abnormality in any of the structures of the LFU can disrupt the normal tear film and the ocular surface and result in DED. Thus, it is important to understand the anatomy and function of each part of the unit for targeted treatment and disease management. A disruption in this unit may develop from aging, decrease in supportive factors (e.g. androgen hormones), and ocular surface diseases, due to meibomian gland dysfunction, viral keratitis or other ocular surface infections, and systemic inflammatory or autoimmune diseases, such as Sjögren's syndrome and rheumatoid arthritis. Structural abnormalities, such as a pterygium, also prevent the smooth distribution of the tear film and can contribute to the development of DED.

DED can generally be divided into two categories: aqueous tear deficiency and evaporative dry eye, each with several subgroups.[12] Aqueous tear deficiency results from a failure of tear secretion, and can be divided into Sjögren's and non-Sjögren's subtypes. It has been shown to involve, at least in part, T-cell mediated inflammation of the lacrimal gland, resulting in diminished tear production and propagation of inflammatory mediators across the ocular surface. Evaporative dry eye is primarily caused by meibomian gland dysfunction (MGD), but may also result from disorders of enlarged lid aperture, as well as low blink rates.[12] In MGD, changes of nonpolar lipids result in alterations of the secreted meibum and obstruction of the meibomian glands, resulting in tear film instability, rapid tear evaporation, tear hyperosmolarity, and initiation of inflammatory cascades.[17] To complicate matters further, in the majority of patients, the two types of DED co-exist, leading to a mixed phenotype.

2.3. *Pathophysiology of DED*

The core mechanisms of DED are believed to be driven by tear hyperosmolarity, tear film instability, and inflammation. Hyperosmolarity arises as a result of tear evaporation from the exposed ocular surface. Hyperosmolarity then induces a cascade of inflammatory events in the surface epithelial cells, which activates mitogen-activated protein kinases (MAPK). The MAPK signaling pathways then stimulate nuclear factor kappa-light-chain-enhancer of activated B cells (NF-κB) signaling pathways and the production of pro-inflammatory cytokines (e.g., interleukin 1α [IL-1α] and interleukin 1β [IL-1β]; tumor necrosis factor α [TNF-α]) and matrix metalloproteinases (MMP). These inflammatory mediators either arise from or activate inflammatory cells (e.g., antigen presenting cells [APCs], T-cells) on the ocular surface,[18–20] which up-regulate the production of additional pro-inflammatory cytokines.[20] Further, there is evidence that inflammatory events result in apoptosis of surface epithelial cells and goblet cells,[21] leading to reduced mucin levels of MUC5AC (a goblet cell-specific mucin) in DED.[22,23] Regardless of the origin, a self-perpetuating cycle of inflammation ensues that is central to the pathogenesis of DED (Fig. 1).[24]

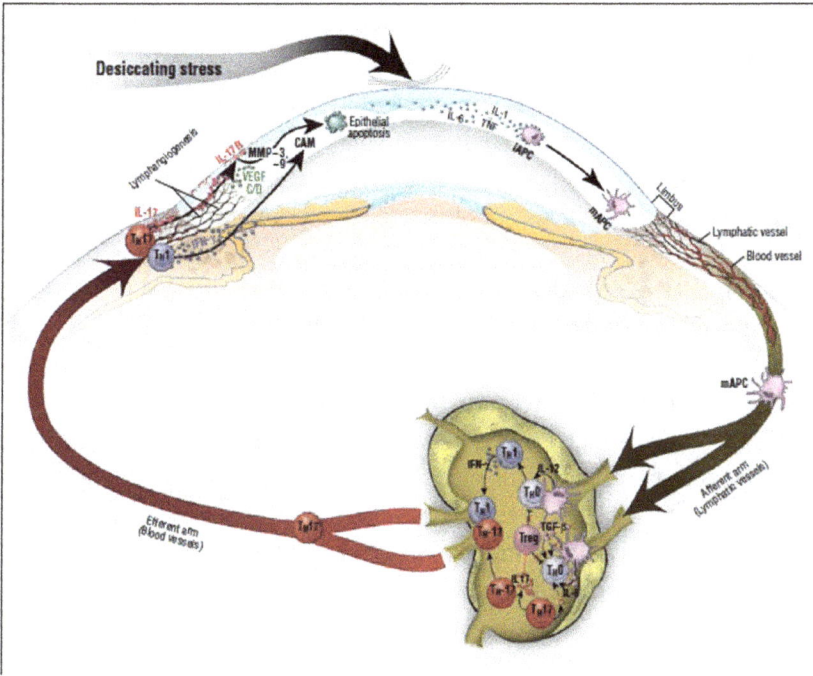

Figure 1. Immunoinflammatory pathways. Desiccating stress induces tear hyperosmolarity, activating intracellular signaling pathways that initiate the production of proinflammatory cytokines (eg, interleukin [IL] 1, tumor necrosis factor [TNF], and IL-6). This proinflammatory milieu facilitates the activation and maturation of immature antigen-presenting cells (iAPC). Mature APCs (mAPC) migrate through the afferent lymphatics to draining lymph nodes, where they induce effector helper T cell 1 (TH1) and TH17 cells that subsequently migrate through efferent blood vessels to the ocular surface. The TH17 cells antagonize regulatory T cell functions and lead to further expansion of T effectors in the draining lymph nodes. Effector TH1-secreted interferon (IFN) and TH17-secreted IL-17 exert their pathogenic effects by promoting the production of proinflammatory cytokines, chemokines, matrix metalloproteinases (e.g., MMP-3 and MMP-9), cell adhesion molecules (CAM), and prolymphangiogenic molecules (vascular endothelial growth factor [VEGF] D and VEGF-C) that facilitate the infiltration of pathogenic immune cells, leading to further damage of the ocular surface. IL-17R indicates IL-17 receptor; TGF, transforming growth factor. (With permission from Archives of Ophthalmology and the American Medical Association on December 11, 2013 (20))

Additionally, tear film instability can be initiated by a number of other ocular, environmental and systemic conditions, including MGD, xerophthalmia, ocular allergies, contact lens wear, dietary consumption of a high ratio of omega-6 to omega-3 essential fatty acids, cigarette smoking, prolonged use of video displays, diabetes mellitus and long term use of medications with topical preservatives such as benzalkonium chloride.[12] Medical conditions such as post-traumatic stress disorder (odds ratio 1.97, 95% CI 1.75–2.23), sleep apnea (odds ratio 2.20, 95% CI 1.91–2.46), depression (odds ratio 1.91, 95% CI 1.73–2.10), and thyroid disease (OR 1.81, 95% CI 1.46–2.26) have been shown to increase risk of DED.[5] History of cigarette smoking and the presence of a pterygium were also found to be independent risk factors.[1] In a Japanese population, low body mass index, contact lens use, and hypertension were risk factors for men. Whereas, contact lens use, myocardial infarction, angina and visual display terminal use were risk factors for women and body mass index was a preventative factor for women.[4] However, irrespective of etiology, DED is associated with inflammation of the ocular surface, which then causes surface damage and further exacerbation of DED.

3. Potential Targets for DED

3.1. *Tear deficiency or increased evaporation*

Until recently, DED was considered to be due to deficiency or evaporation of tears and its therapy was aimed at symptomatic treatment by lubricating and hydrating the ocular surface. Therefore, ocular lubricants remain a mainstay of DED therapy. They act by various mechanisms, such as reducing hypertonicity and improvement of ocular surface wetting,[25] supplementing the lipid layer and preventing evaporation of tears,[26] or supplementation of the mucin layer.[27] The difficulty with ocular lubricants, however, is that most of the formulations have preservatives, which can by themselves exacerbate ocular surface irritation with frequent use.[28] This has necessitated the use of single-use preservative-free vials. They are inconvenient to use, require frequent dosing, and often have only a short duration of symptom relief. In addition, they can blur the vision, especially when in the form of a gel. Reports have also shown that artificial tears lose their efficacy over time. A 2008 Gallup study found that two-thirds (67%; n = 705) of the patients with DED were using artificial tears at initiation of the study, but the dissatisfaction level with tear use more than doubled from 4% (n = 363) to 10% (n = 472) over 6 years (29).

3.2. Inflammation

Inflammation is well established as part of the pathophysiology of DED via several different mechanisms.[20] As discussed above, elevated tear osmolarity can result in the production of pro-inflammatory mediators, such as cytokines, chemokines and MMPs, via the MAPK signaling pathways.[30] These mediators promote epithelial cell damage, thus inducing the formation and activation of additional inflammatory mediators, and further exacerbating surface inflammation.[31-34] In addition, they promote the activation and migration of antigen presenting cells (APCs). APCs are involved in the activation and expansion of T cells, which also invade the ocular surface and produce additional pro-inflammatory mediators.[35,36]

Cytokines that are consistently reported as elevated in the tears of patients with DED include IL-1, IL-6, and TNF.[37-42] Elevated levels of IL-1, IL-6, TNF, and TGF-β1 are seen in conjunctival epithelium as well.[41,53] Additional isolated cytokines on the ocular surface include IL-2, IL-4, IL-5, IL-10, and IFN-gamma.[37] An increased activity of chemokines is also evident in both clinical and animal models of DED.[37-40] Chemokine IL-8 (CXCL8) is consistently elevated in the tear film of patients with DED and CXCL9, CXCL10, CXCL11 are increased as well.[37-43.] Under hyperosmolar stress, corneal epithelial cells will produce MMP-1, MMP-3, MMP-9, and MMP-13 and elevated levels of MMP-9 have been identified in patients with dry eyes.[44-47]

This cycle of inflammation provides a promising target to restore ocular surface health for therapy of DED. Currently, cyclosporine and corticosteroids are used to treat DED, and work by suppressing inflammation. However, they have limited use due to their safety and side effect profiles. Therefore, currently extensive research is directed at identifying new anti-inflammatory therapies with improved efficacy and safety profiles. The success of cyclosporine has made inflammatory mediators promising targets for the treatment of DED. Positive results have been reported with various therapeutic agents targeting mediators such as CCR2, IL-17,[48–50] and several others. In addition, dietary supplements that have anti-inflammatory effects such as certain fatty acids are being evaluated and used for dry eye therapy.[51,52] Further, novel drug delivery systems that increase the drug concentration on the ocular surface are currently under investigation.

3.3. Mucin secretion

Mucin secretagogues are molecules that increase secretion of mucins from goblet cells. The normal tear film contains a layer of aqueous mucin-containing gel. These mucins both have lubricant and defense functions on the ocular surface. The ocular surface epithelium expresses several different mucins. The goblet cells in conjunctiva secrete the gel forming mucin MUC5AC, wheras the stratified epithelium produces the membrane-spaning mucins MUC1 and MUC4.[53,54] MUC2 may also be secreted by the conjunctival epithelium, but at lower levels than the others.[55] Corneal epithelium produces the membrane spanning mucins MUC1, MUC4, and MUC16.[54,56–58] Ocular surface injury can alter the quality and quantity of mucins secreted and cause a reduction in the density of goblet cells.[59] Since the mucins are involved in retention of the aqueous layer, disruption of mucins can further exacerbate DED. Mucin instillations in DED subjects have shown therapeutic effects.[60] Therefore, drugs that increase mucin concentration or replace mucins have been shown to be effective in treating DED. For example, Rebamipide and Diquafasol sodium are mucin secretagogues that have shown efficacy in the treatment of DED and will be discussed in more detail later in the chapter.[61–66]

3.4. Autologous serum tears

Autologous serum tears (AST) drops are hemoderivative products of the patients' own blood. They are a mixture of intracellular and extracellular compounds that include those that are essential for proliferation, differentiation, and maturation of normal ocular surface epithelium such as epidermal growth factor, platelet growth factors, vitamin A, transforming growth factor-β (TGF-β), fibronectin, nerve growth factor, and other cytokines. Many of these compounds are found in the normal tear film. Thus, AST drops are being used for the treatment of severe DED, persistent epithelial defects, neurotrophic keratopathy, and recurrent corneal erosions.[67] By providing substrates for epithelialization and nerve survival, they have proven useful in healing epithelial defects, closing wounds, regaining corneal sensitivity, and reducing recurrences of erosions.[68] Although the drops have been in use for about 30 years.[69] they have only recently been applied for patients with DED and are continually being studied to evaluate their therapeutic effects and optimal protocol for preparation and treatment dosing. Further studies will be discussed later in the chapter.

3.5. *Hormonal mechanisms*

Hormones play a role in ocular surface homeostasis and function through androgen and estrogen receptors. Androgen receptors are present in the meibomian glands of humans (70, 71). A possible mechanism of androgen effects is the association of androgen to the synthesis of TGF-β and reduction in IL-1β and TNF-α in lacrimal glands, which contributes to tear secretion.[72] As for estrogen, its function within meibomian glands and on the ocular surface is not completely understood. It is still not known whether estrogen excess or deficiency, androgen deficiency, or an imbalance between the two affect ocular surface dysfunction. Several studies have shown correlations between the levels of these hormones and tear production, tear film osmolarity and dry eye symptoms. Therefore, further research regarding this topic may provide more opportunities for drug targets and more information regarding disease mechanisms.

4. Current Status of Ocular Drugs and Therapies

Current treatment strategies include artificial tears and other lubricating supplements, punctual plugs, moisture chamber spectacles, contact lenses and anti-inflammatory drugs (e.g., cyclosporine and corticosteroids). Other potential medications are currently used in clinical practice, but are still being extensively studied. The treatment options will be discussed below.

4.1. Stepwise approach from dry eye workshop report

The 2007 DEWS report classified DED into four severity categories.[2] (Table 1). Treatment recommendations by severity level are presented in Table 2.[12] A stepladder approach is applied with conservative management in mild DED, and with increased severity or inadequate response to treatment, the next level of treatment alternatives is recommended.

4.2. Ocular lubricants

One of the first steps of treatment for DED is to replace the patient's tears with artificial tear ophthalmic drops. Ideally, ocular lubricants should improve ocular lubrication as well as decrease evaporation. The main components of artificial tear preparations contain cellulose ethers, carbomers, polyvinyl alcohol, polyvinyl pyrrolidones, or sodium hyaluronate.[73] The majority of the preparations also include preservatives, including benzalkonium chloride (BAK), purite, glycerol, sodium perborate, or polyquarternium (PQ-1); however, these can be irritating to certain patients and therefore preservative-free options with single-use vials are available as well and recommended for more frequent use. Other tear

Table 1. Dry Eye Workshop (DEWS) dry eye severity categories.

Severity Level	1	2	3	4
Symptoms	Mild to moderate	Mild to moderate	Severe	Extremely severe
Conjunctival signs	Mild to moderate	Staining	Staining	Scarring
Corneal Staining		Mild punctate staining	Marked punctate staining, central staining, filamentary keratitis	Severe staining, corneal erosions

Table 2. Treatment recommendations based of severity score from the International Dry Eye Workshop (DEWS) in 2007.

Level 1 Severity (select single option or combination of below)
Simple education/environmental/dietary modifications
Avoidance of medications possibly causing dry eye (when possible)
Artificial tears
Eye warming/lid margin cleansing

Level 2 Severity (in addition to level 1, select a single option or a combination of below)
Topical anti-inflammatory agents
Tetracyclines
Tear secretogogues
Moist chamber spectacles

Level 3 Severity (in addition to level 2, select a single option or a combination of below)
Autologous serum
Punctum cauterization
Contact lenses

Level 4 Severity (in addition to level 3, select a single option or a combination of below)
Systemic anti-inflammatory agents
Surgical alternatives (tarsorrhaphy, amniotic/mucous membrane transplants, salivary gland transplantation)

---

solutions include lipid-containing formulations due to the thought that a lipid would stabilize tears and decrease evaporation as well as friction between the lid and ocular surface.[74,75] FreshKote® (Focus Labs, North Little Rock, Arkansas) contains a combination of all tear components, including polyvinylalcohol and polyvinylpyrrollidone, as well as Amisol® Clear which is intended to stabilize the lipid layer. A cellulose ophthalmic insert (Lacrisert®; Valeant Ophthalmics, New Jersey) is also available and for moderate to severe dry eye and can be inserted into the inferior cul-de-sac once daily for symptom relief. The list of available tear formulations are presented in Table 3.

The use of tears supplements has a number of limitations. Although tear supplements can minimize patients' symptoms and alter the composition of the tears in DED, they do not address the underlying etiology of the condition; neither do punctual plugs, contact lenses, or moisture chamber spectacles. The dosing schedule often requires frequent application and patients often complain of only a short time of symptom relief with each

Table 3. Available artificial tear formulations.

Artificial Tear Components	Name	Company
Carboxymethycellulose base tears	Refresh	Allergan
	Thera Tears	Advanced Vision Research
Hydroxypropylmethylcellulose based artificial tears	Tears Naturale	Alcon
	BionTears	Alcon
	Gen Teal	Novartis
Hydroxypropyl guar based artificial tears	Systane	Alcon
	BionTears	Alcon
	Gen Teal	Novartis
Sodium hyaluronate based artificial tears	Blinktears	AMO
	Blink Contacts	AMO
	AquifyComfort	CIBA
	Hyalein	Santen
Polyvinylalcohol based artificial tears	Murine tears	Murine EyeCare
	Tears again	OcuSoft
	Hypotears	Novartis
Oil based artificial tears	Soothe XP	Bausch&Lomb
	Castor oil	
Propylene glycol, Hydroxypropyl-guar with micro-emulsion of oil eye drop	Systane Balance	Alcon
Polyvinylalcohol and polyvinylpyrrollidone artificial tears	FreshKote	Focus Labs
Hydroxypropyl cellulose ophthalmic insert	Lacrisert	Valeant ophthalmics

use. In addition, it is very difficult to reproduce the natural tears that are made up of complex composition.

4.3. *Anti-inflammatory drugs*

4.3.1. *Cyclosporine A (Restasis®)*

One of the anti-inflammatory agents used for the treatment of DED is cyclosporine A (CsA), which mediates its actions by binding to a specific cytosolic protein, cyclophilin, and inhibiting T-cell activities, such as the release of inflammatory cytokines including IL-2 and interferon

(IFN)-γ. In a randomized, multi-center, double-masked, parallel group, dose-response controlled Phase II clinical trial of topical CsA, four different concentrations of CsA (0.05%, 0.1%, 0.2%, or 0.4%) were evaluated in a twice daily dosing regimen in 129 patients for 12 weeks compared to 33 patients receiving vehicle treatment. In a subset of 90 patients with moderate-to-severe DED, CsA was found to significantly decrease conjunctival staining, superficial punctate keratitis, and ocular irritation as well as dryness symptoms. Although there was no clear dose-response relationship, CsA 0.1% produced the most consistent improvement in evaluated end points and CsA 0.05% showed improvement in patients' symptoms of DED. There were no significant adverse effects, microbial overgrowth, and increased risk of ocular infection in any treatment group. Therefore, the study concluded that 0.1% and 0.05% are the most appropriate formulations for future clinical studies.[76]

A two-center, randomized Phase III clinical trial on CsA in 877 moderate-to-severe DED patients with two different concentrations of CsA (0.05% and 0.1%) showed that treatment with CsA resulted in significantly greater improvements than vehicle in corneal staining and Schirmer's wetting test values. The CsA 0.05% dosing showed significantly greater improvements of DED, including blurred vision, need for concomitant tears, and the physician's evaluation of the patients' response to treatment.[77] Additionally, there was no dose-response effect and both doses of CsA exhibited excellent safety profiles.

Further, Toker and colleagues reported additional beneficial effects of 0.05% topical CsA treatment on corneal and conjunctival sensitivity. A total of 37 patients with DED were treated with CsA 0.05% twice a day and were evaluated at 1, 3, and 6 months. After treatment with topical CsA, statistically significant improvements were observed in corneal sensitivity ($p < 0.0001$) and symptom scores.[78] Moreover, Pflugfelder and co-workers showed that eyes treated with 0.05% CsA had an approximately 200% increase in conjunctival goblet cell density.[79]

Studies have also shown a decreased expression of human leukocyte antigen DR (HLA-DR), apoptosis markers, and IL-6 by conjunctival epithelial cells.[80,81] Furthermore, cyclosporine-treated eyes have shown a shift in the numbers of CD3-, CD4-, and CD8-positive T lymphocytes in the conjunctiva, whereas vehicle-treated eyes showed an increase in these markers.[82] There was also a significant decrease in the number of cells expressing CD11a and HLA-DR, indicating less activation of APCs in vehicle-treated eyes.

Although CsA has shown significant effect in improving DED, there are limitations to its use. For example, not all patients respond well to the treatment of CsA. Additionally, the manufacturer noted that the medication may need to be used for at least 30 days before the therapeutic benefit is observed. With this finding and notable side effects that include burning, stinging, and conjunctival hyperemia, poor patient compliance and therefore poor efficacy is an issue.[83]

4.3.2. Corticosteroids

Corticosteroids are an effective anti-inflammatory agent in the treatment of DED as well. The immunosuppressive effects of corticosteroids are due to nonspecific inhibition of several aspects of the inflammatory response, including inhibition of the activity of transcription factors, such as activator protein-1 (AP-1) and nuclear factor κB (NF-κB), that activate pro-inflammatory genes. Thirty-two patients in an open-label, randomized study received flurometholone plus artificial tear substitutes for DED and experienced lower symptom severity scores and lower rose bengal and fluorescein staining than patients receiving artificial tears plus flurbiprofen or artificial tears alone.[84] Marsh and colleagues reported that in 21 patients with Sjögren's syndrome, use of topical non-preserved methylprednisolone decreased levels of the chemotactic cytokine IL-8 in the conjunctival epithelium and was efficacious for the treatment of severe aqueous deficiency refractory to preservative-free lubricants and punctual occlusion.[85] Additionally, a double-masked, randomized study of 64 patients with keratoconjunctivitis sicca and delayed tear clearance found that loteprednol etabonate 0.5% ophthalmic suspension used four times daily for 4 weeks was more effective than vehicle in improving signs and symptoms.[86] Occasionally in some patients with significant inflammatory disease such as in Sjogren's syndrome, systemic steroids may be more effective for symptom control.[87,88]

The limitations of topical corticosteroid therapy are an increased risk of infection, elevated intraocular pressure, and posterior subcapsular cataracts.[89,90] Therefore, corticosteroids are more appropriate for pulse therapy to control acute exacerbations and not for long-term treatment of DED. After the acute stage is under control, patients should be switched to a low dose and/or transitioned to another means of managing their symptoms with less ocular side effects.

4.4. *Dietary supplementation*

Essential fatty acids are biologically necessary fatty acids that must be ingested. Humans require two essential fatty acids for optimal health, omega-3 (α-linoleic acid) and omega-6 (linoleic acid) fatty acids. Essential fatty acids are the precursors to eicosanoids (prostaglandins, prostacyclins, thromboxanes, and leukotrienes) that modulate immune responses. Omega-3 fatty acids are generally classified as anti-inflammatory fatty acids and function by blocking the production of pro-inflammatory eicosanoids and cytokines.[20, 91–93] Omega-3 fatty acids have been used in the treatment of immune-mediated disorders, including Sjögren's syndrome. However, studies in the treatment of DED have conflicting results. Nevertheless, the majority of the available evidence shows that administration of essential fatty acids, particularly omega-3 fatty acids, can lessen the severity of DED.[51,52,94–97]

Milanjovic and co-workers have shown that women with higher omega-3 fatty acid intake (>5–6 tuna servings per week as opposed to <1) had 68% lower prevalence of DED.[94] In a prospective, placebo-controlled randomized trial of 26 patients with aqueous-deficient DED, study group patients receiving tablets containing linoleic (LA, 28.5 mg) and gamma-linoleic acid (GLA, 15 mg) twice daily for 45 days had statistically significant changes in dry eye symptoms, lissamine green staining and ocular surface inflammation as compared to the placebo group. Ocular surface inflammation was measured based on HLA-DR expression. Percentage of HLA-DR expression in the conjunctival cells decreased from $58.5 \pm 14.1\%$ to $41.3 \pm 18.9\%$ in the treated group and from 61.4 ± 21.9 to $58.0 \pm 13.3\%$ in the placebo group. There was no statistically significant difference between groups for tear break up time (TBUT) and the Schirmer's I test.[51]

A randomized, double-masked study evaluating 61 patients with symptoms of signs of MGD found that oral omega-3 fatty acids at 1.5 grams per day may be beneficial for the treatment of MGD mainly by improving tear stability. After 3 months of evaluation, the mean Ocular Surface Disease Index (OSDI), TBUT, lid margin inflammation, and meibomian gland expression were improved from baseline ($p < 0.01$, $p < 0.001$, $p < 0.0001$, $p < 0.0001$, respectively) in the group using omega-3 supplementation versus the group with just lid hygiene only.[98] Another study also showed improvement in ocular symptoms and corneal surface smoothness when using gamma-linolenic acid (GLA) and omega-3 fatty acids in patients with keratoconjunctivitis sicca over 6 months.[99] Kangari et al. found significant improvement in the mean TBUT, OSDI, and Schimer's test in patients treated with omega-3 daily for one month ($p < 0.001$, $p = 0.004$, $p = 0.033$, respectively) dosed at 180 mg eicosapentaenoid acid (EPA) and 120 mg docosahexaenoic acid (DHA) twice daily.[100]

4.5. *Other ocular drugs and therapies for dry eye disease*

Topical acetylcysteine is a mucolytic agent that is sometimes used in patients with dense mucus accumulation or filamentary keratitis.[101] It works by breaking disulfide bonds within mucus, which then liquefies it. It is most often used as an inhalational bronchial mucolytic agent for patients with dense pulmonary mucus, such as in patients with cystic and pulmonary fibrosis. Acetylcysteine is not commercially available in a topical ophthalmic formulation,[102] but inhalational acetylcysteine has been used in diluted forms for off-label use.

Tetracyclines provide a therapeutic benefit in DED likely related to their anti-inflammatory and lipid regulating properties, more than their antimicrobial effects. The use of tetracyclines will be discussed in greater detail later in the chapter.

There are also new procedures that are available to target patients with DED, especially those with a component of MGD. Lipiflow Theramal Pulsation System® (TearScience, North Carolina) is a technology designed to unblock meibomian glands by applying both localized heat and recurrent pressure on the eyelids. The theory behind the technology is that unblocking the glands will restore natural oil secretion and therefore a healthy tear film. It has shown success in the treatment of MGD and dry eye symptoms and signs.[103] Intense pulse light (IPL) treatment is another available option, which was originally developed for use in dermatology for patients with acne and rosacea.[104] It involves powerful bursts of light at specific wavelengths that induce changes within the surface of the skin and may be beneficial to meibomian gland function. Finally, intraductal meibomian gland probing also has been shown to be effective in patients with MGD and associated DED.[105]

5. Ongoing Clinical Trials and Potential Future Therapies (Table 4)

5.1. *Mucin secretagogues*

5.1.1. *Rebamipide*

Rebamipide is a quinolone derivative with mucin secretagogue activity. It is an oral therapeutic agent effective in the treatment of gastric ulcers and gastritis in humans by increasing mucin levels.[106] It has also been shown to increase the production of mucin-like substances in the cornea and conjunctiva of a rabbit model in which mucin was decreased by N-acetylcysteine.[61] In a randomized, double-masked, multi-center, placebo-controlled, parallel-group, dose-response Phase II study.[63] on 308 DED patients, rebamipide showed significant dose-responsive efficacy in improvement of ocular staining scores, TBUT, and patients' symptoms after 4 weeks of treatment. It was relatively well tolerated with the most frequently observed adverse events being dysgeusia, eye irritation, and nasopharyngitis.[63] Another more recent study.[62] evaluated 154 patients with DED treated with 2% rebamipide four times daily for 52 weeks. For all signs and symptoms, the scores were significantly improved at 2 weeks compared to baseline ($p < 0.001$) and improved with each follow-up visit up to the 52-week period.[62]

5.1.2 *Diquafosol tetrasodium*

Diquafosal tetrasodium is a mucin secretagogue, a topical P2Y2 receptor agonist, and a member of the adenosine triphosphate receptor family.

Table 4 Ongoing clinical trials and potential future therapies.

Class	Drug	Company	Phase of Development	Mechanism of Action
Anti-inflammatory and Immunomodulators	Cyclosporine A (Cyclokat)	Novagali Pharma (Santen)	Phase III clinical trial	Immunosuppresant
				T-cell inhibitor
				Calcineurin inhibitor
	Resolvin E 1 (RvE1)	Resolvyx Pharmaceuticals	Phase I clinical trial	Possible anti-inflammatory
		Celtic Therapeutics	No development reported	
	Lifitegrast (SAR1118)	Sunesis	Discontinued	Lymphocyte function-associated molecule inhibitor
		SARCode	Phase III clinical trial	
	Dexamethasone phosphate (EGP-437)	EyeGate Pharma	Phase III clinical trial	Glucocorticoid agonist
				Arachidonic acid inhibitor
				Corticosteroid agonist
	CF-101	Can-Fite	Phase III clinical trial	Adenosine A3 receptor agonist
		BioPharma	Phase I clinical trial	Granulocyte simulating factor agonist
		Seikagaku Kwang Dong	Preclinical	
	Tofacitinib (CP-690,550)	Pfizer	Launched	Janus kinase 3 inhibitor
		Takeda	Phase II clinical trial	Janus kinase 1 hinibitor
				Disease modifying anti-rheumatic drug immunosuppressant
				Tyrosine kinase inhibitor
				MAPK inhibitor
	Tacrolimus	Isotechnika Pharma	Phase I clinical trial	Calcineurin inhibitor
		Lux Biosciences	Phase I clinical trial	

Category	Drug	Company	Status	Mechanism
	Thymosin B4 RegeneRx (RGN-259)	RegeneRx Biopharmaceuticals	Phase II clinical trial	Thymosin fraction B4 agonist
		Sigma-Tau	Phase II clinical trial	MMP-9 inhibitor; Metalloproteinase-1 inhibitor
		Lee's Pharmaceuticals	Preclinical	Angiogenesis stimulant Anti-inflammatory; Wound healing; Anti-apoptotic; Inhibition of NF-κB
	Topical infliximab	EyeGate Pharma	Animal research	TNF-alpha inhibitor; Anti-inflammatory
	Anakinra/IL-1 antagonist	Amgen Inc	Pilot studies	Recombinant human IL-1Ra; Anti-inflammatory
Mucin secretagogues	Rebamipide	Otsuka	Launched	Oxygen scavenger
		Acucela	Phase III clinical trial	Mucus protecting agent
		Novartis	No development reported	Prostaglandin synthase stimulant
	Diquafosol tetrasodium	Allergan	No development reported	Purinoreceptor P2Y2 agonist
		Santen	Launched	
		Kissei	Discontinued	
		Hoffman-La Roche	Discontinued	
Other	MIM-D3	Mimetogen Pharmaceuticals Inc	Phase II clinical trial	Mimetic of nerve growth factor; Maintaining ocular surface

Activation of the Gq protein-couple P2Y2 receptor results in non-glandular secretion of mucins and water via chloride channel activation. In addition to secreting fluid and mucins, it can potentially restore conjunctival goblet cells and stimulate lipid production from meibocytes.[65] Results from clinical trials indicate that topical diquafosol (1% and 3%) can lead to dose-dependent improvements in ocular surface staining in DED as compared to the placebo.[64] and that the 3% strength is more effective than the 1% formulation. In addition, improvements in staining scores found in the Phase II and Phase III studies were maintained for up to 52 weeks without deterioration, thereby demonstrating the continuous efficacy of diquafosol over a long period.[64] In another study, diquafosol tetrasodium was effective in improving the objective signs and subjective symptoms in patients where sodium hyaluronate monotherapy was insufficient and thus may be used for additive therapeutic effects in such patients.[66]

5.2. Ocular lubricants

5.2.1 Sodium hyaluronate

Hyaluronic acid in various formulations continues to be evaluated in several studies. It has been shown to possess anti-inflammatory, wound-healing, and water retention properties and thus has a beneficial role in DED by increasing ocular wettability.[107] Sodium hyaluronate drops improve tear film stability.[108] and may be more effective than carboxymethylcellulose in improving symptoms of DED.[109] A hypotonic 0.18% sodium hyaluronate drop has demonstrated statistically significant improvement in DED, both in symptom frequency score and fluorescein staining score.[110] Several other Phase II/III trials have been completed or are currently underway by Alcon, River Plate, and Allergan.

5.3. Anti-inflammatory antibiotics

Tetracyclines have a therapeutic effect in DED mainly due to their anti-inflammatory and lipid-regulating properties, rather than for their antimicrobial effects. They have shown immunomodulatory properties at submicrobial doses. They exert anti-inflammatory effects due to inhibition of MAPK, MMPs, cytokines, lymphocytes, and neutrophils. They also have anti-angiogenic and anti-apoptotic properties.[111] Doxycycline has been shown to inhibit c-Jun N-terminal kinase and extracellular signaling in epithelial cells of the ocular surface exposed to hyperosmolar stress, down-regulating the expression of CXCL8 and pro-inflammatory cytokines IL-1b and TNF-a.[112] Doxycyline also inhibits activity of MMPs and supports ocular surface integrity.[111,113] Minocycline inhibits expression of cell-associated pro-inflammatory molecules, including MHC class II.[114] The anti-inflammatory mechanisms of azithromycin are not completely understood, but it has been demonstrated that azithromycin can block the activation of NF-κB, leading to a decrease in inflammatory cyctokines such as IL-6 and IL-8.[115]

Though the most common route of intake is oral, topical formulations are being studied. In an experimental DED model, it was shown that liposomal-bound topical doxycycline may be useful in increasing bioavailability of doxycycline.[116] Topical azithromycin 1% was shown to be effective in treating DED associated with MGD/blepharitis and contact lens wear.[117–119] Additionally, pulsed oral azithromycin therapy has shown clinical efficacy in the treatment of posterior blepharitis.[120] The anti-inflammatory benefits of orally administered tetracycline derivatives have been used in the treatment of chronic immune-mediated diseases, including DED secondary to ocular rosacea and blepharitis.[121–124] However, larger studies are needed to clearly outline the safety and efficacy of these drugs in DED and also to address the possibility of increased microbial resistance with long-term use of topical antibiotics.

5.4. *Autologous*

5.4.1. *Serum tears*

Autologous serum tears are generated from a patient's own serum have been used in the treatment of severe DED. Studies have shown that autologous serum (AST) drops were more effective than artificial tears in terms of TBUT, corneal staining, and symptom scores.[125,126] However, there are concerns with AST such as the risk of microbial growth.[127] and risks associated with periodic blood draws. Although AST drops contain antimicrobial agents such as immunoglobulins and lysozyme, they also contain high protein content, which increases the risk of microbial growth.[127] As a precaution, AST drops may be diluted to 20%; however, concentrations between 20–100% have been used. Several small, randomized studies investigating autologous serum tears versus unpreserved eye drops or other conventional treatments have shown autologous serum tears to be effective in improving symptom and signs of DED associated with Sjögren's and non-Sjögrens dry eye and post-LASIK dry eye. However, a recent Cochrone-based review of the available studies concluded that there was still inconsistency in the results of various trials and a well-planned, large, high-quality clinical trial is warranted to determine the true benefits of serum tears.[128]

To address the concerns of blood draws, cord blood serum drops (prepared from donor umbilical cord blood serum) and allogenic drops (from related donors) have been studied as alternatives. In patients with chronic graft-versus-host disease, allogenic serum drops have shown to decrease symptom scores, tear osmolarity, and corneal staining, and increase goblet cell density and TBUT significantly after 4 weeks of treatment.[129] In another study on 30 patients (17 were graft-versus-host disease and 13 were Sjogren's syndrome), cord blood serum drops significantly improved corneal sensitivity, Schirmer's scores, TBUT, tear osmolarity, and cytology scores for inflammation, and reduced corneal epithelial damage.[130] Therefore, allogenic and cord blood serum drops pose as potential alternatives for patients who are unable to or are uncomfortable with AS drops. However, issues such as the optimal dilution of serum needed, correct storage and preservation to maintain efficacy of the biologically active constituents, and the potential of transmission of infections through blood products may hinder the routine use of these drops for the treatment of DED.

5.4.2. Autologous plasma

Autologous platelet-rich plasma (PRP) has shown effectiveness in both wound healing and tissue regeneration. It provides a higher concentration of growth factors and cell adhesion molecules by concentrating platelets in a small volume of plasma.[131] Therefore, it has also been studied in its healing effects on the corneal surface in the treatment of DED. One study evaluated 18 patients with symptomatic DED treated with topical PRP and followed for 1 month. Symptoms improved significantly in 89% of patients and improved conjunctival hyperemia and corneal fluorescein staining was also observed.[132] Another study found good results in healing of epithelial defects with autologous plasma rich in growth factors.[133]

5.5. Hormonal therapy

Androgenic steroid therapy for the treatment of DED has been of increased interest. Androgens seem to have some immunosuppressive effects, while estrogens have been associated with progression or involvement in autoimmune disorders. The effects of hormone therapy on tear function are likely the result of changes on both the lacrimal and meibomian glands. Systemic androgen hormone therapy, in murine models of Sjögren's syndrome, decreased the size and number of lacrimal gland lymphocytic foci and reduced lymphocytic infiltration.[12] Androgens immunosuppressive effects may be the result of an increase in TGF-beta, a strong anti-inflammatory cytokine, and a reduction in IL-1β and TNF-α. Previously shown, topically applied 0.03% testosterone improves meibomian gland secretions and relieves symptoms of discomfort over 6 months of use.[134] Additional topical preparations of androgen steroid hormones are under evaluation in randomized clinical trials.

A randomized, double-blind, placebo controlled, crossover study.[135] examined 66 postmenopausal women with DED for the efficacy of an oral phytoestrogen supplement (Lacrisek®; BIOOS Italia Srl, Italy) and placebo tablet. Phytoestrogens are non-steroidal plant compounds that are structurally and functionally similar to 17-β estradiol, and produce effects similar to estrogen on estrogen receptors. The study concluded that: (1) there is a significant inverse correlation between sex steroid levels and tear osmolarity; (2) phytoestrogen significantly lowered tear osmolarity and improved Schirmer's test results; and (3) symptoms improved as measured by OSDI. No adverse events were reported.

However, estrogen-related studies have contradicted each other. A randomized, double-blind, parallel-group study.[136] in 42 postmenopausal women studying the efficacy of hormone therapy for 3 months, specifically 17-β estradiol combined with medroxyprogesterone acetate, found no significant support for hormone therapy as there was no statistically significant difference between the treatment group and control group in terms of tear secretion, TBUT, and corneal thickness. While a greater number of patients reported improvement in symptoms in the treatment group, the difference between treatment and control groups was not significant.

5.6. *Anti-inflammatory drugs and immunomodulators*

5.6.1. *Cyclokat (Nova22007)*

Cyclokat is a topical cyclosporine, which differs from Restasis® in two ways: it has a higher concentration of cyclosporine (0.1 vs 0.05%), and includes a novel drug delivery system in the form of cationic emulsion of cyclosporine A, based on Novagali s Novasorb® technology. The positively charged emulsion electrostatically adheres to the negatively charged epithelial layer of the eye, and may thereby improve ocular absorption.[137]

A recent study.[138] evaluated the ocular and systemic distribution of cyclosporine A in rabbits after instillation of Restasis® (anionic cyclosporine A emulsion) twice daily or NOVA22007 (cationic cyclosporine A emulsion) daily for 10 days. Higher concentrations of CsA were delivered to the cornea with NOVA22007 0.1% or 0.05% compared to Restasis®. Importantly, systemic distribution after repeated instillations was low and comparable between all the emulsions.[138]

A six-month Phase III, multicenter, randomized, controlled double-masked trial of Cyclokat versus vehicle, evaluating 492 patients with moderate to severe DED showed statistically significant improvements in Cyclokat-treated patients over vehicle in mean corneal fluorescein staining change from baseline to month 1 (-0.77 vs. 0.52, $p = 0.002$), month 3 (-0.92 vs. -0.70, $p = 0.030$), and month 6 (-1.05 vs -0.82, $p = 0.009$), and these better outcomes seemed to be enhanced in patients with more severe keratitis.[139] In a recent Phase II, multicenter, randomized, double-masked, vehicle controlled study of 132 patients receiving Cylcokat applied daily for over three months, Cyclokat demonstrated significant treatment effect on multiple efficacy variables for both signs and symptoms at months 1 and 3.[140] These results are currently unpublished. Another Phase III, multicenter, double-masked, two parallel arm, vehicle controlled, 6-month study with 6-months of follow up is currently ongoing and results are pending.[141]

5.6.2 Resolvin E1 (RvE1)

Resolvin E1 (RvE1) is an endogenous mediator of immune response that is derived from the lipoxygenation of the essential dietary omega-3 fatty acids, docosahexaenoic acid, and eicosapentaenoic acid.[142] They have been shown to be effective immunomodulators in preclinical models of colitis,[143] arthritis,[144] and airway inflammation.[145] In animal models, these omega-3 derivatives have been shown to reverse corneal epithelial damage associated with DED, increase tear flow, promote healthy epithelium, and decrease cyclooxygenase-2 expression and macrophage infiltration.[146] RvE1 improved the outcome measures of corneal staining and goblet cell density in a murine model.[147] A Phase II clinical trial is testing the synthetic analog of RvE1 (RX-10045, Auven Therapeutics) for the treatment of chronic DED. Preliminary data of a randomized, placebo-controlled, trial with 232 patients showed dose-dependent and statistically significant improvements in DED over 28 days in patients treated with RX-10045. However, final results are still pending.

5.6.3. Lifitegrast (SAR 1118)

SAR 1118 is a novel investigational lymphocyte function-associated antigen-1 (LFA-1) antagonist engineered for topical ophthalmic delivery.[148, 149] LFA-1 on the surface of T cells binds to intercellular adhesion molecule-1 (ICAM-1) on endothelial, epithelial, and immune function cells and is a critical step in T-cell trafficking in both normal immune response and inflammation. Thus, it has been proposed that blockade of LFA-1/ICAM-1 interaction may confer a therapeutic benefit in patients with

DED, preventing T-cell recruitment and T-cell mediated inflammation and thus aiding the recovery of the ocular surface.

A recent study evaluated the potential of Lifitegrast (Shire, Lexington, MA) to block corneal inflammation in a murine model. Results showed a decrease in neutrophil recruitment in the cornea and decreased microbial-induced inflammation.[150] Clinical trials in humans have shown a good safety and tolerability profile.[151,152] An 84-day multicenter, prospective, double-masked, placebo-controlled trial of 230 subjects with DED randomized to receive SAR 1118 (0.1, 1.0 or 5.0%) or placebo drops twice daily showed dose-dependence and statistically significant improvements in corneal staining score, total ocular surface disease index (OSDI), and visual-related function OSDI scores for SAR 111. Tear production and symptom improvements were observed as early as day 14. Lifitegrast was well tolerated and without serious ocular adverse events.[149]

OPUS-1 was a Phase III prospective, randomized, double-masked, placebo-controlled, parallel arm, multicentral clinical trial assessing the efficacy and safety of Lifitegrast 5.0% compared to placebo on the treatment of dry eye disease. It found that Lifitegrast significantly reduced corneal fluorescein staining and conjunctival lissamine stainging as well as improved symptoms of ocular discomfort and eye dryness over 84 days.[153] OPUS-2 is an ongoing Phase III study that is still pending published results, however, Shire (biopharmaceutical company, Lexington, MA) has announced results that suggest that there is symptom improvement over the trial period in patients using Lifitegrast, however, the medication did not meet the other endpoints that were seen in OPUS-1. OPUS-2 is different than OPUS-1 in that patients in OPUS-2 have had a recent history of artificial tear use. SONATA is another study evaluating specifically the safety of Lifitegrast over an extended time period. So far, OPUS-2 has not shown evidence of any serious side effects. The most common treatment related adverse events have been dysguesia, instillation site irritation, and instillation site reaction.

5.6.4. EGP-437

EGP-437 is a 40 mg/mL dexamethasone phosphate solution, delivered to the ocular tissues via a novel ocular iontophoresis platform, the EyeGate

II system® (Eyegate Pharmaceuticals, Inc, Waltham, MA, USA).[154] Iontophoresis involves placing drug molecules in a small electric field created on the ocular surface, which may increase the mobility of the drug molecules and lead to a higher concentration of the drug in the tissues than achieved by eye drops. In preclinical studies on rabbit eye models, iontophoresis of EGP-437 was shown to deliver significantly higher aqueous humor drug concentration levels than topical or intravenous administration,[155] and led to significantly better DED signs within 2 days of application.

Another recent study,[156] evaluated the toxicokinetics and tolerability of EGP-437 delivered to the eyes of rabbits by transscleral iontophoresis biweekly for 24 consecutive weeks at different designated dosages. The results of the study suggest that repeated doses of EGP-437 may be safe for use as a treatment of ocular inflammatory disorders that require prolonged or repeated steroid therapy.[156]

In a Phase II prospective, single-center, double-masked randomized controlled trial using controlled adverse environment of 103 subjects with DED, iontophoresis of EGP-437 showed statistically significant improvement in signs and symptoms of DED at various time points over a 3-week study duration.[154] However, treatment related adverse events were experienced by 87% of patients (consistent across all treatment groups). Though most adverse events were mild and no severe adverse events were observed, 2.4% of one of the active groups had lenticular opacities, vitreous floaters, or corneal deposits, which were not seen in the placebo group. A Phase III clinical trial of EGP-437 in 193 DED subjects has been completed though results are yet to be published.

5.6.5. *CF101*

CF101, generically known as IB-MECA, is an adenosine receptor agonist shown in preclinical and clinical studies to mediate a marked anti-inflammatory effect in a variety of systemic inflammatory diseases.[157–160] A Phase II, randomized, controlled, double-masked clinical trial concluded that 1-mg doses of CF101 twice daily for 12 weeks induced a statistically significant improvement in the corneal staining, TBUT, and tear meniscus height in patients with moderate to severe DED. The adverse events most frequently reported were constipation, headache, palpitations, itching, abdominal pain, arthralgia, myalgia, fatigue, and dry mouth but reportedly these were mild and the drug was well tolerated overall.[161] A Phase III clinical trial sponsored by Can-Fite BioPharma is currently recruiting patients.[162]

5.6.6. *Topical tofacitinib (CP-690,550)*

Topical tofacitinib is a Janus kinase inhibitor that has demonstrated a trend for improving both signs and symptoms of DED in both Phase I and II trials. Tofacitinib has a functional cellular selectivity for JAK1 and JAK3 over JAK2.[163] JAK signaling is critical for immune cell activation, proliferation, proinflammatory cytokine production, and cytokine signaling.[164] Due to the association of DED and inflammatory processes, Pfizer Inc. conducted Phase I/II prospective, randomized, double-masked, multicenter, vehicle- and comparator-controlled clinical trials to assess its efficacy in DED (NCT00784719). The groups received tofacitinib (0.0003%, 0.001%, 0.003%, or 0.005% two times daily or 0.005% once daily), or the comparator (0.05% CsA) or vehicle twice daily for 8 weeks. All doses of tofacitinib eye drops demonstrated a trend toward improving both signs and symptoms of moderate to severe DED, with a reasonably safe profile. However, there was no clear dose response or efficacy observed. A substudy did show decreased conjunctival cell surface HLA-DR expression and decrease in the levels of pro-inflammatory cytokines in tears and inflammatory markers such as MMP-3, MMP-9, IL-1β, IL-15, IL-17A, and IL-12p70 during the 8-week period.

5.6.7. *Thymosin β4 (RGN-259)*

Thymosin β4/RGN-259 (RegeneRx Biopharmaceuticals Inc., Rockville, MD) is an intracellular polypeptide comprising 43 amino acids.[24,165] Thymosin β4 has both anti-inflammatory and wound-healing properties.[166] that are thought to be an ideal combination for the treatment of DED.[165] In the cornea, thymosin β4 has demonstrated anti-apoptotic activity and the ability to up-regulate antioxidant enzymes, resulting in protection against oxidative damage in human corneal epithelial cells (167, 168). There has also been discussion around thymosin β4 and its ability to inhibit the

NF-κB-mediated inflammatory pathways in the cornea.[169] NF-κB has also been discussed as a potential target for treatment of DED.

One Phase II study reported was a double-masked, single-center study with 70 patients who were randomized to receive either 0.1% RGN-259 or placebo (preservative-free eye drops) twice daily for 28 days. RGN-259 caused significant improvements in ocular surface discomfort and corneal staining, and was safe and well tolerated.[170] Another Phase II study was a double-masked, vehicle-controlled, physician-sponsored trial for treating severe DED. Nine patients were treated with RGN-259 or a vehicle control six times daily for 28 days. Preliminary results showed that RGN-259 met efficacy objectives, with statistically significant improvements in signs and symptoms of DED compared to vehicle control at various time intervals.[171]

5.6.8. *Topical tacrolimus*

Topical tacrolimus is a calcineurin inhibitor that has some clinical evidence of good efficacy in DED and was evaluated for tolerability in a Phase I study (Lux BioSciences, Jersey City, NJ, LX-214 [voclosporin].[172] In ophthalmology, systemic use of tacrolimus is already well established in the treatment of immune-mediated diseases, uveitis,[173,174] DED secondary to graft-versus-host disease, corneal transplants, and ocular pemphigoid. It is also used topically as an ointment, to treat ocular allergies, especially atopic blepharoconjunctivitis.[175–177] Its use for DED is only in the early stages of evaluation, but its use has been described in animals.[178]

A recent study evaluated use of topical tacrolimus 0.03% in sixteen eyes with Sjögren's syndrome DED. The results showed improved fluorescein and rose bengal staining scores after 14, 28, and 90 days of treatment, improved average Schirmer's I test after 90 days, and improved average TBUT after 28 and 90 days of treatment.[179]

5.7. Biologics

5.7.1. *Topical infliximab*

Topical infliximab is a TNF-α inhibitor that has shown promising results in murine models of DED.[180] Experimental DED was induced in C57BL/6 mice and the mice were treated with different concentrations of balanced salt solution or infliximab. Mice treated with different concentrations of infliximab (0.01% or 0.1%) showed improvement in tear volume and corneal smoothness compared to controls. At both concentrations, infliximab-treated mice showed lower levels of conjunctival inflammatory cytokines (IL-1B, IL6, IL-17 and interferon-γ), decreased staining intensity of TNF-α, and increased density of goblet cells.[180]

5.7.2. IL-1 Receptor antagonist

Anakinra, an IL-1 receptor antagonist (Kineret; Amgen Inc, Thousand Oaks, CA), is a recombinant version of human IL-1Rα approved for treatment of rheumatoid arthritis.[181] Anakinra has also been used off label for the treatment of many other conditions that involve IL-1-mediated inflammation.[182] A recent study.[183] showed that topical anakinra was effective in treating DED in an animal model. IL-1 has previously been implicated in the immunopathogenic mechanisms of DED-associated ocular inflammation. A recent study.[184] using topical 2.5% anakinra for 12 weeks for the treatment of DED showed the treatment to be well tolerated and safe with a significant reduction in symptoms and corneal epitheliopathy. After 12 weeks of therapy, participants receiving anakinra 2.5% achieved a 46% reduction in their mean corneal fluorescein staining score ($p = 0.12$ compared with vehicle and $p < 0.001$ compared to baseline), compared to patients receiving vehicle who achieved a 19% reduction. In addition, at week 12, patients receiving anakinra 2.5% had a significant reduction in symptoms at 30% compared to a 5% reduction of symptoms in patients receiving vehicle.[184] Also, Eleven Biotherapeutics (Cambridge, MA) presented clinical data that demonstrated that their IL-1 receptor inhibitory (EBI-005) had significant improvement in signs (OSDI and corneal fluorescein staining) and symptoms from baseline ($p < 0.001$). Patients using EBI-005 also used less rescue artificial tear drops and the medication was well-tolerated.[185]

5.8. MIM-D3

MIM-D3 is a small-molecular mimetic of nerve growth factor (NGF) that is being investigated by Mimetogen Pharmaceuticals Inc (Gloucester,

MA). Various studies have reported that NGF plays an important role in maintaining and regenerating the ocular surface.[186-188] Studies have shown that topical application of 1% MIM-D3 increased the glycoconjugate concentration in tears and reduced corneal epithelial damage in a rat model of DED.[189]

Mimetogen conducted a Phase II clinical trial in which a total of 150 patients were randomized to receive 1% or 5% MIM-D3 or placebo two times daily for 28 days. The preliminary results demonstrated statistically significant improvements in the signs and symptoms of DED with both doses of MIM-D3 along with good safety and tolerability profiles.[189]

6. Conclusions

DED is one of the most common ocular morbidities with a significant impact on a patient's quality of life and on health care costs. Though there are several treatment options available, they are limited by issues of efficacy, side effects, high frequency of application, and compliance to treatment, and only one drug (Restasis®) is FDA approved. Thus, there is an unmet need to identify novel therapeutic targets for the treatment of DED. The growing knowledge of the pathophysiology of DED and the disruptions of the tear film has driven the development of many new molecules that target core mechanisms and pathways in DED. These include strategies such as inhibiting inflammation on the ocular surface, supplementing the tear film with substances that increase tear film stability and thus prevent ocular surface damage, stimulating secretion of mucins, or correcting underlying hormonal imbalances. Ultimately the goal of drug discovery in DED is to break the cycle of DED and prevent recurrence of symptoms by restoring and strengthening the normal ocular surface.

7. References

1. Lee, A.J., Lee, J., Saw, S.M., Gazzard, G., Koh, D., Widjaja, D., *et al.* Prevalence and risk factors associated with dry eye symptoms: A population based study in Indonesia. *Br J Ophthalmol* **86**(12), 1347–1351 (2002).
2. Uchino, M., Dogru, M., Uchino, Y., Fukagawa, K., Shimmura, S., Takebayashi, T., *et al.* Japan Ministry of Health study on prevalence of dry

eye disease among Japanese high school students. *Am J Ophthalmol* **146**(6), 925–929 e2 (2008).

3. Uchino, M., Schaumberg, D.A., Dogru, M., Uchino, Y., Fukagawa, K., Shimmura, S., *et al.* Prevalence of dry eye disease among Japanese visual display terminal users. *Ophthalmology* **115**(11), 1982–1988 (2008).

4. Uchino, M., Nishiwaki, Y., Michikawa, T., Shirakawa, K., Kuwahara, E., Yamada, M., *et al.* Prevalence and risk factors of dry eye disease in Japan: Koumi study. *Ophthalmology* **118**(12), 2361–2367 (2011).

5. Galor, A., Feuer, W., Lee, D.J., Florez, H., Carter, D., Pouyeh, B., *et al.* Prevalence and risk factors of dry eye syndrome in a United States veterans affairs population. *Am J Ophthalmol* **152**(3), 377–384 e2 (2011).

6. Schaumberg, D.A., Sullivan, D.A., Buring, J.E., Dana, M.R. Prevalence of dry eye syndrome among US women. *Am J Ophthalmol* **136**(2), 318–326 (2003).

7. Miljanovic, B., Dana, M.R., Sullivan, D.A., Schaumberg, D.A. Prevalence and risk factors for dry eye syndrome among older men in the United States [ARVO #4293]. *ARVO*, (2007).

8. Friedman, N.J. Impact of dry eye disease and treatment on quality of life. Curr *Opin Ophthalmol* **21**(4), 310–316 (2010).

9. Buchholz, P., Steeds, C.S., Stern, L.S., Wiederkehr, D.P., Doyle, J.J., Katz L.M., *et al.* Utility assessment to measure the impact of dry eye disease. *Ocul Surf* **4**(3), 155–161 (2006).

10. Schiffman, R.M., Walt, J.G., Jacobsen, G., Doyle, J.J., Lebovics, G., Sumner W. Utility assessment among patients with dry eye disease. *Ophthalmology* **110**(7), 1412–1419 (2003).

11. Yu, J., Asche, C.V., Fairchild, C.J. The economic burden of dry eye disease in the United States: A decision tree analysis. *Cornea* **30**(4), 379–387 (2011).

12. The definition and classification of dry eye disease: report of the Definition and Classification Subcommittee of the International Dry Eye WorkShop. *Ocul Surf* **5**(2), 75–92 (2007).

13. Nagyova, B., Tiffany, J.M. Components responsible for the surface tension of human tears. *Curr Eye Res* **19**(1), 4–11 (1999).

14. Glasson, M.J., Stapleton, F., Keay, L., Sweeney, D., Willcox M.D. Differences in clinical parameters and tear film of tolerant and intolerant contact lens wearers. *Invest Ophthalmol Vis Sci* **44**(12), 5116–5124 (2003).

15. Begley, C.G., Chalmers, R.L., Abetz, L., Venkataraman, K., Mertzanis, P., Caffery, B.A., *et al.* The relationship between habitual patient-reported symptoms and clinical signs among patients with dry eye of varying severity. *Invest Ophthalmol Vis Sci* **44**(11), 4753–4761 (2003).

16. Pflugfelder, S.C. Tear dysfunction and the cornea: LXVIII Edward Jackson Memorial Lecture. *Am J Ophthalmol* **152**(6), 900–909 e1 (2011).
17. Bron, A.J., Tiffany, J.M. The contribution of meibomian disease to dry eye. *Ocul Surf* **2**(2), 149–165 (2004).
18. Luo, L., Li, D.Q., Corrales, R.M., Pflugfelder, S.C. Hyperosmolar saline is a proinflammatory stress on the mouse ocular surface. *Eye Contact Lens* **31**(5), 186–193 (2005).
19. De Paiva, C.S., Corrales, R.M., Villarreal, A.L., Farley, W.J., Li, D.Q., Stern, M.E., *et al.* Corticosteroid and doxycycline suppress MMP-9 and inflammatory cytokine expression, MAPK activation in the corneal epithelium in experimental dry eye. *Exp Eye Res* **83**(3), 526–535 (2006).
20. Stevenson, W., Chauhan, S.K., Dana, R. Dry eye disease: An immune-mediated ocular surface disorder. *Arch Ophthalmol* **130**(1), 90–100 (2012).
21. Yeh, S., Song, X.J., Farley, W., Li, D.Q., Stern, M.E., Pflugfelder, S.C. Apoptosis of ocular surface cells in experimentally induced dry eye. *Invest Ophthalmol Vis Sci* **44**(1), 124–129 (2003).
22. Zhao, H., Jumblatt, J.E., Wood, T.O., Jumblatt, M.M. Quantification of MUC5AC protein in human tears. *Cornea* **20**(8), 873–877 (2001).
23. Argueso, P., Balaram, M., Spurr-Michaud, S., Keutmann, H.T., Dana, M.R., Gipson, I.K. Decreased levels of the goblet cell mucin MUC5AC in tears of patients with Sjogren syndrome. *Invest Ophthalmol Vis Sci* **43**(4), 1004–1111 (2002).
24. Goldstein, A.L., Hannappel, E., Kleinman, H.K. Thymosin beta4: Actin-sequestering protein moonlights to repair injured tissues. *Trends Mol Med* **11**(9), 421–429 (2005).
25. Brignole, F., Pisella, P.J., Dupas, B., Baeyens, V., Baudouin, C. Efficacy and safety of 0.18% sodium hyaluronate in patients with moderate dry eye syndrome and superficial keratitis. *Graefes Arch Clin Exp Ophthalmol* **243**(6), 531–538 (2005).
26. Scaffidi, R.C., Korb, D.R. Comparison of the efficacy of two lipid emulsion eyedrops in increasing tear film lipid layer thickness. *Eye Contact Lens* **33**(1), 38–44 (2007).
27. Benelli, U. Systane lubricant eye drops in the management of ocular dryness. *Clin Ophthalmol* **5**, 783–790 (2011).
28. Foulks, G.N. BAK to basics. *Ocul Surf* **9**(3), 139 (2011).
29. The Gallup Organization, Inc. The 2008 gallup study of dry eye sufferers. *Multi-Sponser Surveys*, Inc; Princeton, NJ: (2008).
30. Li, D.Q., Luo, L., Chen, Z., Kim, H.S., Song, X.J., Pflugfelder, S.C. JNK and ERK MAP kinases mediate induction of IL-1beta, TNF-alpha and IL-8

following hyperosmolar stress in human limbal epithelial cells. *Exp Eye Res* **82**(4), 588–596 (2006).

31. Chen, Y.T., Nikulina, K., Lazarev, S., Bahrami, A.F., Noble, L.B., Gallup, M., *et al.* Interleukin-1 as a phenotypic immunomodulator in keratinizing squamous metaplasia of the ocular surface in Sjogren's syndrome. *Am J Pathol* **177**(3), 1333–1343 (2010).

32. De Paiva, C.S., Villarreal, A.L., Corrales, R.M., Rahman, H.T., Chang, V.Y., Farley, W.J., *et al.* Dry eye-induced conjunctival epithelial squamous metaplasia is modulated by interferon-gamma. *Invest Ophthalmol Vis Sci* **48**(6), 2553–2560 (2007).

33. Luo, L., Li, D.Q., Pflugfelder, S.C. Hyperosmolarity-induced apoptosis in human corneal epithelial cells is mediated by cytochromec and MAPK pathways. *Cornea* **26**(4), 452–460 (2007).

34. Yeh, S., Song, X.J., Farley, W., Li, D.Q., Stern, M.E., Pflugfelder, S.C. Apoptosis of ocular surface cells in experimentally induced dry eye. *Invest Ophthalmol Vis Sci* **44**(1), 124–129 (2003).

35. El Annan, J., Chauhan, S.K., Ecoiffier, T., Zhang, Q., Saban, D.R., Dana, R. Characterization of effector T cells in dry eye disease. *Invest Ophthalmol Vis Sci* **50**(8), 3802–3807 (2009).

36. De Paiva, C.S., Chotikavanich, S., Pangelinan, S.B., Pitcher, J.D., 3rd, Fang, B., Zheng, X., *et al.* IL-17 disrupts corneal barrier following desiccating stress. *Mucosal immunology* **2**(3), 243–253 (2009).

37. Massingale, M.L., Li, X., Vallabhajosyula, M., Chen, D., Wei, Y., Asbell, P.A. Analysis of inflammatory cytokines in the tears of dry eye patients. *Cornea* **28**(9), 1023–1027 (2009).

38. Pflugfelder, S.C., Jones, D., Ji, Z., Afonso, A., Monroy, D. Altered cytokine balance in the tear fluid and conjunctiva of patients with Sjogren's syndrome keratoconjunctivitis sicca. *Curr Eye Res* **19**(3), 201–211 (1999).

39. Yoon, K.C., De Paiva, C.S., Qi, H., Chen, Z., Farley, W.J., Li, D.Q., *et al.* Expression of Th-1 chemokines and chemokine receptors on the ocular surface of C57BL/6 mice: Effects of desiccating stress. *Invest Ophthalmol Vis Sci* **48**(6), 2561–2569 (2007).

40. El Annan, J., Goyal, S., Zhang, Q., Freeman, G.J., Sharpe, A.H., Dana, R. Regulation of T-cell chemotaxis by programmed death-ligand 1 (PD-L1) in dry eye-associated corneal inflammation. *Invest Ophthalmol Vis Sci* **51**(7), 3418–3423 (2010).

41. Lam, H., Bleiden, L., de Paiva, C.S., Farley, W., Stern, M.E., Pflugfelder, S.C. Tear cytokine profiles in dysfunctional tear syndrome. *Am J Ophthalmol* **147**(2), 198-205 e1 (2009).

42. Enriquez-de-Salamanca, A., Castellanos, E., Stern, M.E., Fernandez, I., Carreno, E., Garcia-Vazquez, C., *et al.* Tear cytokine and chemokine analysis and clinical correlations in evaporative-type dry eye disease. Molecular vision **16**, 862–873 (2010).

43. Yoon, K.C., Park, C.S., You, I.C., Choi, H.J., Lee, K.H., Im, S.K., *et al.* Expression of, CX.L., -10, -11, and CXCR3 in the tear film and ocular surface of patients with dry eye syndrome. *Invest Ophthalmol Vis Sci* **51**(2), 643–650 (2010).

44. Solomon, A., Dursun, D., Liu, Z., Xie, Y., Macri, A., Pflugfelder SC. Pro- and anti-inflammatory forms of interleukin-1 in the tear fluid and conjunctiva of patients with dry-eye disease. *Invest Ophthalmol Vis Sci* **42**(10), 2283–2292 (2001).

45. Li, D.Q., Chen, Z., Song, X.J., Luo, L., Pflugfelder, S.C. Stimulation of matrix metalloproteinases by hyperosmolarity via a JNK pathway in human corneal epithelial cells. *Invest Ophthalmol Vis Sci* **45**(12), 4302–4311 (2004).

46. Chotikavanich, S., de Paiva, C.S., Li de, Q., Chen, J.J., Bian, F., Farley, W.J., *et al.* Production and activity of matrix metalloproteinase-9 on the ocular surface increase in dysfunctional tear syndrome. *Invest Ophthalmol Vis Sci* **50**(7), 3203–3209 (2009).

47. Acera, A., Rocha, G., Vecino, E., Lema, I., Duran, J.A. Inflammatory markers in the tears of patients with ocular surface disease. *Ophthalmic Res* **40**(6), 315–321 (2008).

48. Goyal, S., Chauhan, S.K., Zhang, Q., Dana, R. Amelioration of murine dry eye disease by topical antagonist to chemokine receptor 2. *Arch Ophthalmol* **127**(7), 882–887 (2009).

49. Ecoiffier, T., El Annan, J., Rashid, S., Schaumberg, D., Dana, R. Modulation of integrin alpha4beta1 (VLA-4) in dry eye disease. *Arch Ophthalmol* **126**(12), 1695–1659 (2008).

50. Chauhan, S.K., El Annan, J., Ecoiffier, T., Goyal, S., Zhang, Q., Saban, D.R., *et al.* Autoimmunity in dry eye is due to resistance of Th17 to Treg suppression. *J Immunol* **182**(3), 1247–1252 (2009).

51. Barabino, S., Rolando, M., Camicione, P., Ravera, G., Zanardi, S., Giuffrida, S., *et al.* Systemic linoleic and gamma-linolenic acid therapy in dry eye syndrome with an inflammatory component. *Cornea* **22**(2), 97–101 (2003).

52. Wojtowicz, J.C., Butovich, I., Uchiyama, E., Aronowicz, J., Agee, S., McCulley J.P. Pilot, prospective, randomized, double-masked, placebo-controlled clinical trial of an omega-3 supplement for dry eye. *Cornea* **30**(3), 308–314 (2011).

53. Inatomi, T., Spurr-Michaud, S., Tisdale, A.S., Zhan, Q., Feldman, S.T., Gipson I.K. Expression of secretory mucin genes by human conjunctival epithelia. *Invest Ophthalmol Vis Sci* **37**(8), 1684–1692 (1996).

54. Inatomi, T., Spurr-Michaud, S., Tisdale, A.S., Gipson, I.K. Human corneal and conjunctival epithelia express MUC1 mucin. *Invest Ophthalmol Vis Sci* **36**(9), 1818–1827 (1995).

55. McKenzie, R.W., Jumblatt, J.E., Jumblatt, M.M. Quantification of MUC2 and MUC5AC transcripts in human conjunctiva. *Invest Ophthalmol Vis Sci* **41**(3), 703–708 (2000).

56. Gipson, I.K., Argueso, P. Role of mucins in the function of the corneal and conjunctival epithelia. *Int rev Cytology* **231**, 1–49 (2003).

57. Govindarajan, B., Gipson, I.K. Membrane-tethered mucins have multiple functions on the ocular surface. *Exp Eye Res* **90**(6), 655–663 (2010).

58. Blalock, T.D., Spurr-Michaud, S.J., Tisdale, A.S., Gipson, I.K. Release of membrane-associated mucins from ocular surface epithelia. *Invest Ophthalmol Vis Sci* **49**(5), 1864–1871 (2008).

59. Gipson, I.K., Hori, Y., Argueso, P. Character of ocular surface mucins and their alteration in dry eye disease. *Ocul Surf* **2**(2), 131–148 (2004).

60. Shigemitsu, T., Shimizu, Y., Ishiguro K. Mucin ophthalmic solution treatment of dry eye. *Adv Exp Med Biol* **506**(Pt A), 359–362 (2002).

61. Urashima, H., Okamoto, T., Takeji, Y., Shinohara, H., Fujisawa, S. Rebamipide increases the amount of mucin-like substances on the conjunctiva and *cornea* in the N-acetylcysteine-treated in vivo model. *Cornea* **23**(6), 613–619 (2004).

62. Kinoshita, S., Awamura, S., Nakamichi, N., Suzuki, H., Oshiden, K., Yokoi, N., *et al.* A Multicenter, Open-Label, 52-Week Study of 2% Rebamipide (OPC-12759) Ophthalmic Suspension in Patients with Dry Eye. *Am J Ophthalmol* (2013).

63. Kinoshita, S., Awamura, S., Oshiden, K., Nakamichi, N., Suzuki, H., Yokoi, N., *et al.* Rebamipide (OPC-12759) in the treatment of dry eye: A randomized, double-masked, multicenter, placebo-controlled phase II study. *Ophthalmology* **119**(12), 2471–2478 (2012).

64. Matsumoto, Y., Ohashi, Y., Watanabe, H., Tsubota, K., Diquafosol Ophthalmic Solution Phase 2 Study G. Efficacy and safety of diquafosol ophthalmic solution in patients with dry eye syndrome: A Japanese phase 2 clinical trial. *Ophthalmology* **119**(10), 1954–1960 (2012).

65. Nichols, K.K., Yerxa, B., Kellerman DJ. Diquafosol tetrasodium: A novel dry eye therapy. *Expert Opin Investig Drugs* **13**(1), 47–54. (2004).

66. Kamiya, K., Nakanishi, M., Ishii, R., Kobashi, H., Igarashi, A., Sato, N., *et al.* Clinical evaluation of the additive effect of diquafosol tetrasodium on sodium hyaluronate monotherapy in patients with dry eye syndrome: a prospective, randomized, multicenter study. *Eye (Lond)* **26**(10), 1363–1368 (2012).

67. Geerling, G., Maclennan, S., Hartwig D. Autologous serum eye drops for ocular surface disorders. *Br J Ophthalmol* **88**(11), 1467–1474 (2004).

68. Matsumoto, Y., Dogru, M., Goto, E., Ohashi, Y., Kojima, T., Ishida, R., *et al.* Autologous serum application in the treatment of neurotrophic keratopathy. *Ophthalmology* **111**(6), 1115–1120 (2004).

69. Tsubota, K., Goto, E., Fujita, H., Ono, M., Inoue, H., Saito, I., *et al.* Treatment of dry eye by autologous serum application in Sjogren's syndrome. *Br J Ophthalmol* **83**(4), 390–395 (1999).

70. Rocha, E.M., Wickham, L.A., da Silveira, L.A., Krenzer, K.L., Yu, F.S., Toda, I., *et al.* Identification of androgen receptor protein and 5alpha-reductase mRNA in human ocular tissues. *Br J Ophthalmol* **84**(1), 76–84 (2000).

71. Auw-Haedrich, C., Feltgen, N. Estrogen receptor expression in meibomian glands and its correlation with age and dry-eye parameters. *Graefes Arch Clin Exp Ophthalmol* **241**(9), 705–709 (2003).

72. Sullivan, D.A., Wickham, L.A., Rocha, E.M., Kelleher, R.S., da Silveira, L.A., Toda I. Influence of gender, sex steroid hormones, and the hypothalamic-pituitary axis on the structure and function of the lacrimal gland. *Adv Exp Med Biol* **438**, 11–42 (1998).

73. Calonge M. The treatment of dry eye. *Surv Ophthalmol* **45** Suppl 2, S227–239 (2001).

74. Rieger G. Lipid-containing eye drops: A step closer to natural tears. *Ophthalmologica* **201**(4), 206–212 (1990).

75. Tiffany J.M. Lipid-containing eye drops. *Ophthalmologica* **203**(1), 47–49 (1991).

76. Stevenson, D., Tauber, J., Reis, B.L. Efficacy and safety of cyclosporin A ophthalmic emulsion in the treatment of moderate-to-severe dry eye disease: a dose-ranging, randomized trial. The Cyclosporin A Phase 2 Study Group. *Ophthalmology* **107**(5), 967–974 (2000).

77. Sall, K., Stevenson, O.D., Mundorf, T.K., Reis, B.L. Two multicenter, randomized studies of the efficacy and safety of cyclosporine ophthalmic emulsion in moderate to severe dry eye disease. CsA Phase 3 Study Group. *Ophthalmology* **107**(4), 631–639 (2000).

78. Toker, E., Asfuroglu, E. Corneal and conjunctival sensitivity in patients with dry eye: The effect of topical cyclosporine therapy. *Cornea* **29**(2), 133–140 (2010).
79. Pflugfelder, S.C., De Paiva, C.S., Villarreal, A.L., Stern M.E. Effects of sequential artificial tear and cyclosporine emulsion therapy on conjunctival goblet cell density and transforming growth factor-beta2 production. *Cornea* **27**(1), 64–69 (2008).
80. Brignole, F., Pisella, P.J., De Saint Jean, M., Goldschild, M., Goguel, A., Baudouin, C. Flow cytometric analysis of inflammatory markers in KCS: 6-month treatment with topical cyclosporin A. *Invest Ophthalmol Vis Sci* **42**(1), 90–95 (2001).
81. Turner, K., Pflugfelder, S.C., Ji, Z., Feuer, W.J., Stern, M., Reis, B.L. Interleukin-6 levels in the conjunctival epithelium of patients with dry eye disease treated with cyclosporine ophthalmic emulsion. *Cornea* **19**(4), 492–496 (2000).
82. Kunert, K.S., Tisdale, A.S., Stern, M.E., Smith, J.A., Gipson, I.K. Analysis of topical cyclosporine treatment of patients with dry eye syndrome: Effect on conjunctival lymphocytes. *Arch Ophthalmol* **118**(11), 1489–496 (2000).
83. Ridder, W.H., 3rd. Ciclosporin use in dry eye disease patients. *Expert Opin Pharmacother* **9**(17), 3121–3128 (2008).
84. Avunduk, A.M., Avunduk, M.C., Varnell, E.D., Kaufman, H.E. The comparison of efficacies of topical corticosteroids and nonsteroidal anti-inflammatory drops on dry eye patients: a clinical and immunocytochemical study. *Am J Ophthalmol* **136**(4), 593–602 (2003).
85. Marsh, P., Pflugfelder, S.C. Topical nonpreserved methylprednisolone therapy for keratoconjunctivitis sicca in Sjogren syndrome. *Ophthalmology* **106**(4), 811–816 (1999).
86. Pflugfelder, S.C., Maskin, S.L., Anderson, B., Chodosh, J., Holland, E.J., De Paiva, C.S., *et al.* A randomized, double-masked, placebo-controlled, multicenter comparison of loteprednol etabonate ophthalmic suspension, 0.5%, and placebo for treatment of keratoconjunctivitis sicca in patients with delayed tear clearance. *Am J Ophthalmol* **138**(3), 444–457 (2004).
87. Cordero-Coma, M., Anzaar, F., Sobrin, L., Foster, C.S. Systemic immuno-modulatory therapy in severe dry eye secondary to inflammation. *Ocul Immunol Inflamm* **15**(2), 99–104 (2007).
88. Tabbara, K.F., Frayha, R.A. Alternate-day steroid therapy for patients with primary Sjogren's syndrome. Annals of *ophthalmology* **15**(4), 358–361 (1983).

89. Ramsell, T.G., Trillwood, W., Draper, G. Effects of prednisolone eye drops. A trial of the effects of prednisolone phosphate eye drops on the intra-ocular pressure of normal volunteers. *Br J Ophthalmol* **51**(6), 398–402 (1967).

90. Frandsen E. Glaucoma and posterior subcapsular cataract following topical prednisolone (ultracortenol) therapy. *Acta Ophthalmol (Copenh)* **42**, 108–118 (1964).

91. Rosenberg, E.S., Asbell, P.A. Essential fatty acids in the treatment of dry eye. *Ocul Surf* **8**(1), 18–28 (2010).

92. James, M.J., Gibson, R.A., Cleland, L.G. Dietary polyunsaturated fatty acids and inflammatory mediator production. *Am J Clin Nutr* **71**(1 Suppl), 343S–348S (2000).

93. Endres, S., Ghorbani, R., Kelley, V.E., Georgilis, K., Lonnemann, G., van der Meer, J.W., *et al.* The effect of dietary supplementation with n-3 polyunsaturated fatty acids on the synthesis of interleukin-1 and tumor necrosis factor by mononuclear cells. *N Engl J Med* **320**(5), 265–271 (1989).

94. Miljanovic, B., Trivedi, K.A., Dana, M.R., Gilbard, J.P., Buring, J.E., Schaumberg, D.A. Relation between dietary n-3 and n-6 fatty acids and clinically diagnosed dry eye syndrome in women. *Am J Clin Nutr* **82**(4), 887–893 (2005).

95. Aragona, P., Bucolo, C., Spinella, R., Giuffrida, S., Ferreri, G. Systemic omega-6 essential fatty acid treatment and pge1 tear content in Sjogren's syndrome patients. *Invest Ophthalmol Vis Sci* **46**(12), 4474–4479 (2005).

96. Oxholm, P., Manthorpe, R., Prause, J.U., Horrobin, D. Patients with primary Sjogren's syndrome treated for two months with evening primrose oil. *Scandinavian J Rheumatol* **15**(2), 103–108 (1986).

97. Theander, E., Horrobin, D.F., Jacobsson, L.T., Manthorpe, R. Gammalinolenic acid treatment of fatigue associated with primary Sjogren's syndrome. *Scand J Rheumatol* **31**(2), 72–79 (2002).

98. Olenik, A., Jimenez-Alfaro, I., Alejandre-Alba, N., Mahillo-Fernandez, I. A randomized, double-masked study to evaluate the effect of omega-3 fatty acids supplementation in meibomian gland dysfunction. *Clin Interventions Aging* **8**, 1133–1138 (2013).

99. Sheppard, J.D., Jr., Singh, R., McClellan, A.J., Weikert, M.P., Scoper, S.V., Joly, T.J., *et al.* Long-term supplementation with n-6 and n-3 pufas improves moderate-to-severe keratoconjunctivitis sicca: A randomized double-blind clinical trial. *Cornea* (2013).

100. Kangari, H., Eftekhari, M.H., Sardari, S., Hashemi, H., Salamzadeh, J., Ghassemi-Broumand, M., *et al.* Short-term consumption of oral omega-3 and dry eye syndrome. *Ophthalmology* **120**(11), 2191–2196 (2013).

101. Albietz, J., Sanfilippo, P., Troutbeck, R., Lenton LM. Management of filamentary keratitis associated with aqueous-deficient dry eye. *Optom Vis Sci* **80**(6), 420–430 (2003).
102. Lemp, M.A. Management of dry eye disease. Am J Managed care **14**(3 Suppl), S88–101 (2008).
103. Greiner, J.V. A single LipiFlow(R) Thermal Pulsation System treatment improves meibomian gland function and reduces dry eye symptoms for 9 months. *Curr Eye Res* **37**(4), 272–278 (2012).
104. Mark, K.A., Sparacio, R.M., Voigt, A., Marenus, K., Sarnoff, D.S. Objective and quantitative improvement of rosacea-associated erythema after intense pulsed light treatment. *Dermatol Surg* **29**(6), 600–604 (2003).
105. Wladis, E.J. Intraductal meibomian gland probing in the management of ocular rosacea. *Ophthalmic Plastic Reconstructive sur* **28**(6), 416–418 (2012).
106. Iijima, K., Ichikawa, T., Okada, S., Ogawa, M., Koike, T., Ohara, S., *et al.* Rebamipide, a cytoprotective drug, increases gastric mucus secretion in human: evaluations with endoscopic gastrin test. *Diges Dis and Sci* **54**(7), 1500–1507 (2009).
107. Rah, M.J. A review of hyaluronan and its ophthalmic applications. *Optometry* **82**(1), 38–43 (2011).
108. Yamaguchi, M., Kutsuna, M., Maruo, H., Hara, Y., Uno, T., Kataoka, H., *et al.* [Sustained effects of sodium hyaluronate solution on tear film stability evaluated by Tear Stability Analysis System]. *Nippon Ganka Gakkai zasshi* **115**(2), 134–141 (2011).
109. Dumbleton, K., Woods, C., Fonn, D. An investigation of the efficacy of a novel ocular lubricant. *Eye Contact Lens* **35**(3), 149–155 (2009).
110. Baeyens, V., Bron, A., Baudouin, C., Vismed/Hylovis Study, G. Efficacy of 0.18% hypotonic sodium hyaluronate ophthalmic solution in the treatment of signs and symptoms of dry eye disease. *J Fr Ophtalmol* **35**(6), 412–419 (2012).
111. De Paiva, C.S., Corrales, R.M., Villarreal, A.L., Farley, W.J., Li, D.Q., Stern, M.E., *et al.* Corticosteroid and doxycycline suppress MMP-9 and inflammatory cytokine expression, MAPK activation in the corneal epithelium in experimental dry eye. *Exp Eye Res* **83**(3), 526–535 (2006).
112. Solomon, A., Rosenblatt, M., Li, D., Monroy, D., Ji, Z., Lokeshwar, B.L., *et al.* Doxycycline inhibition of interleukin-1 in the corneal epithelium. *Am J Ophthalmol* **130**(5), 688 (2000).
113. De Paiva, C.S., Corrales, R.M., Villarreal, A.L., Farley, W., Li, D.Q., Stern, M.E., *et al.* Apical corneal barrier disruption in experimental murine dry eye

is abrogated by methylprednisolone and doxycycline. *Invest Ophthalmol Vis Sci* **47**(7), 2847–2856 (2006).

114. Nikodemova, M., Watters, J.J., Jackson, S.J., Yang, S.K., Duncan, I.D. Minocycline down-regulates MHC II expression in microglia and macrophages through inhibition of IRF-1 and protein kinase C (PKC)alpha/betaII. *J Biol Chem* **282**(20), 15208–15216 (2007).

115. Aghai, Z.H., Kode, A., Saslow, J.G., Nakhla, T., Farhath, S., Stahl, G.E., *et al.* Azithromycin suppresses activation of nuclear factor-kappa B and synthesis of pro-inflammatory cytokines in tracheal aspirate cells from premature infants. *Pediatric Res* **62**(4), 483–488 (2007).

116. Shafaa, M.W., El Shazly, L.H., El Shazly, A.H., El gohary, A.A., El hossary, G.G. Efficacy of topically applied liposome-bound tetracycline in the treatment of dry eye model. *Vet Ophthalmol* **14**(1), 18–25 (2011).

117. Veldman, P., Colby, K. Current evidence for topical azithromycin 1% ophthalmic solution in the treatment of blepharitis and blepharitis-associated ocular dryness. *Int Ophthalmol Clin* **51**(4), 43–52 (2011).

118. Nichols, J.J., Bickle, K.M., Zink, R.C., Schiewe, M.D., Haque, R.M., Nichols, K.K. Safety and efficacy of topical azithromycin ophthalmic solution 1.0% in the treatment of contact lens-related dry eye. *Eye Contact Lens* **38**(2), 73–79 (2012).

119. Foulks, G.N., Borchman, D., Yappert, M., Kakar, S. Topical azithromycin and oral doxycycline therapy of meibomian gland dysfunction: a comparative clinical and spectroscopic pilot study. *Cornea* **32**(1), 44–53 (2013).

120. Igami, T.Z., Holzchuh, R., Osaki, T.H., Santo, R.M., Kara-Jose, N., Hida, R.Y. Oral azithromycin for treatment of posterior blepharitis. *Cornea* **30**(10), 1145–1149 (2011).

121. Voils, S.A., Evans, M.E., Lane, M.T., Schosser, R.H., Rapp, R.P. Use of macrolides and tetracyclines for chronic inflammatory diseases. *Ann Pharmacotherapy* **39**(1), 86–94 (2005).

122. Stone, D.U., Chodosh, J. Oral tetracyclines for ocular rosacea: An evidence-based review of the literature. *Cornea* **23**(1), 106–109 (2004).

123. Gilbard, J.P. Dry eye, blepharitis and chronic eye irritation: divide and conquer. *J Ophthalmic Nursing Tech* **18**(3), 109–115 (1999).

124. Bartholomew, R.S., Reid, B.J., Cheesbrough, M.J., Macdonald, M., Galloway, N.R. Oxytetracycline in the treatment of ocular rosacea: A double-blind trial. *Br J Ophthalmol* **66**(6), 386–388 (1982).

125. Urzua, C.A., Vasquez, D.H., Huidobro, A., Hernandez, H., Alfaro, J. Randomized double-blind clinical trial of autologous serum versus artificial tears in dry eye syndrome. *Curr Eye Res* **37**(8), 684–688 (2012).

126. Kojima, T., Ishida, R., Dogru, M., Goto, E., Matsumoto, Y., Kaido, M., *et al.* The effect of autologous serum eyedrops in the treatment of severe dry eye disease: A prospective randomized case-control study. *Am J Ophthalmol* **139**(2), 242–246 (2005).

127. Tananuvat, N., Daniell, M., Sullivan, L.J., Yi, Q., McKelvie, P., McCarty, D.J., *et al.* Controlled study of the use of autologous serum in dry eye patients. *Cornea* **20**(8), 802–806 (2001).

128. Pan, Q., Angelina, A., Zambrano, A., Marrone, M., Stark, W.J., Heflin, T., *et al.* Autologous serum eye drops for dry eye. The Cochrane database of systematic reviews 8:CD009327 (2013).

129. Na, K.S., Kim, M.S. Allogeneic serum eye drops for the treatment of dry eye patients with chronic graft-versus-host disease. *J Ocul Pharmacol Ther* **28**(5), 479–483 (2012).

130. Versura, P., Profazio, V., Buzzi, M., Stancari, A., Arpinati, M., Malavolta, N., *et al.* Efficacy of standardized and quality-controlled cord blood serum eye drop therapy in the healing of severe corneal epithelial damage in dry eye. *Cornea* **32**(4), 412–418 (2013).

131. Alio, J.L., Arnalich-Montiel, F., Rodriguez, A.E. The role of "eye platelet rich plasma" (E-PRP) for wound healing in ophthalmology. *Curr Pharm Biotech* **13**(7), 1257–1265 (2012).

132. Alio, J.L., Colecha, J.R., Pastor, S., Rodriguez, A., Artola, A. Symptomatic dry eye treatment with autologous platelet-rich plasma. *Ophthalmic Res* **39**(3), 124–129 (2007).

133. Lopez-Plandolit, S., Morales, M.C., Freire, V., Etxebarria, J., Duran, J.A. Plasma rich in growth factors as a therapeutic agent for persistent corneal epithelial defects. *Cornea* **29**(8), 843–848 (2010).

134. Schiffman, R.M., Bradford, R., Bunnell, B., *et al.* A multicenter, double-masked, randomized, vehicle-controlled, parallel group study to evaluate the safety and efficacy of testosterone ophthalmic solution in patients with meibomian gland dysfunction. *ARVO* 2006, E-Abstract 5608.

135. Scuderi, G., Contestabile, M.T., Gagliano, C., Iacovello, D., Scuderi, L., Avitabile, T. Effects of phytoestrogen supplementation in postmenopausal women with dry eye syndrome: a randomized clinical trial. *Can J Ophthalmol* **47**(6), 489–492 (2012).

136. Piwkumsribonruang, N., Somboonporn, W., Luanratanakorn, P., Kaewrudee, S., Tharnprisan, P., Soontrapa S. Effectiveness of hormone therapy for treating dry eye syndrome in postmenopausal women: A randomized trial. *J Medical Assoc Thailand Chotmaihet thangphaet* 93(6), 647–652 (2010).

137. Lallemand, F., Daull, P., Benita, S., Buggage, R., Garrigue, J.S. Successfully improving ocular drug delivery using the cationic nanoemulsion, novasorb. *J Drug Deliv* 2012, 604204 (2012).

138. Daull, P., Lallemand, F., Philips, B., Lambert, G., Buggage, R., Garrigue, J.S. Distribution of cyclosporine A in ocular tissues after topical administration of cyclosporine A cationic emulsions to pigmented rabbits. *Cornea* 32(3), 345–354 (2013).

139. Buggage, R.R., Amrane, M., Ismail, D., *et al.* The effect of Cyclokat (Unpreserved 0.% cyclosporine cationic emulsion) on corneal involvement in patietns with moderate to severe dry eye disease participating in a Phase, II.I., multicenter, randomized, controlled, double-masked clinical trial. Eur J Ophthhalmol published online 4/14/2011 11:07:01AM; DOI:10.5301/ EJO.2011.7544 (2001).

140. NOVA22007 0.05% and 0.1% Cyclosporine Versus Vehicle for the Treatment of Dry Eye. Website: http://clinicaltrials.gov/ct2/show/NCT00739349?term= cyclosporine+AND+dry+eye&rank=5 [Accessed on Dec 2013)

141. A multicenter, randomized, double-masked, 2 parallel arm, vehicle con-trolled, 6-month phase III trial with a 6 month follow-up period to evaluate the efficacy and safety of cyclokat® 1mg/ml (ciclosporin/cyclosporine) eye drops, emulsion administered once daily in adult patients with severe dry eye disease. Available from: http://apps.who.int/trialsearch/trial.aspx? trialid=EUCTR2011-000160-97-GB [Accessed Dec 2013].

142. Serhan, C.N., Chiang, N., Van Dyke, T.E. Resolving inflammation: dual anti-inflammatory and pro-resolution lipid mediators. *Nat Rev Immunol* 8(5), 349–361 (2008).

143. Arita, M., Yoshida, M., Hong, S., Tjonahen, E., Glickman, J.N., Petasis, N.A., *et al.* Resolvin E1, an endogenous lipid mediator derived from omega-3 eicosapentaenoic acid, protects against 2,4,6-trinitrobenzene sulfonic acid-induced colitis. *Proc Natl Acad Sci U S A* 102(21), 7671–7676 (2005).

144. Gjorstrup, P., Dubroskiy, A., Dodge, D., *et al.* Resolvin (RvE1) an endoge-nously formed immune modulator attenuates clinical signs of autoimmune disease in the Rat C1A model concurrent with inhibition of T-cell dependent cytokines in mixed cell populations from draining lymph nodes. Presented at: The Association of Research and Vision and Ophthalmology; May 3–7 Fort Lauderdale, FL; A819 (2009).

145. Haworth, O., Cernadas, M., Yang, R., Serhan, C.N., Levy, B.D. Resolvin E1 regulates interleukin 23, interferon-gamma and lipoxin A4 to promote the resolution of allergic airway inflammation. *Nat Immunol* 9(8), 873–879 (2008).

146. Li, N., He, J., Schwartz, C.E., Gjorstrup, P., Bazan, H.E. Resolvin E1 improves tear production and decreases inflammation in a dry eye mouse model. *J Ocul Pharmacol Ther* **26**(5), 431–439 (2010).
147. de Paiva, C.S., Schwartz, C.E., Gjorstrup, P., Pflugfelder, S.C. Resolvin E1 (RX-10001) reduces corneal epithelial barrier disruption and protects against goblet cell loss in a murine model of dry eye. *Cornea* **31**(11), 1299–1303 (2012).
148. Murphy, C.J., Bentley, E., Miller, P.E., McIntyre, K., Leatherberry, G., Dubielzig, R., *et al.* The pharmacologic assessment of a novel lymphocyte function-associated antigen-1 antagonist (SAR 1118) for the treatment of keratoconjunctivitis sicca in dogs. *Invest Ophthalmol Vis Sci* **52**(6), 3174–3180 (2011).
149. Semba, C.P., Torkildsen, G.L., Lonsdale, J.D., McLaurin, E.B., Geffin, J.A., Mundorf, T.K., *et al.* A phase 2 randomized, double-masked, placebo-controlled study of a novel integrin antagonist (SAR 1118) for the treatment of dry eye. *Am J Ophthalmol* **153**(6), 1050–1060 e1 (2012).
150. Sun, Y., Zhang, R., Gadek, T.R., O'Neill, C.A., Pearlman E. Corneal inflammation is inhibited by the LFA-1 antagonist, lifitegrast (SAR 1118*). J Ocul Pharmacol Ther* **29**(4), 395–402 (2013).
151. Paskowitz, D.M., Nguyen, Q.D., Gehlbach, P., Handa, J.T., Solomon, S., Stark, W., *et al.* Safety, tolerability, and bioavailability of topical SAR 1118, a novel antagonist of lymphocyte function-associated antigen-1: A phase 1b study. *Eye (Lond)* **26**(7), 944–949 (2012).
152. Semba, C.P., Swearingen, D., Smith, V.L., Newman, M.S., O'Neill, C.A., Burnier, J.P., *et al.* Safety and pharmacokinetics of a novel lymphocyte function-associated antigen-1 antagonist ophthalmic solution (SAR 1118) in healthy adults. *J Ocul Pharmacol Ther* **27**(1), 99–104 (2011).
153. Sheppard, J.D., Torkildsen, G.L., Lonsdale, J.D., D'Ambrosio, F.A., Jr., McLaurin, E.B., Eiferman, R.A., *et al.* Lifitegrast Ophthalmic Solution 5.0% for Treatment of Dry Eye Disease: Results of the OPUS-1 Phase 3 Study. *Ophthalmology.* 2013.
154. Patane, M.A., Cohen, A., From, S., Torkildsen, G., Welch, D., Ousler, G.W., 3rd. Ocular iontophoresis of EGP 437 (dexamethasone phosphate) in dry eye patients: Results of a randomized clinical trial. *Clin Ophthalmol* **5**, 633–643 (2011).
155. Gungor, S., Delgado-Charro, M.B., Ruiz-Perez, B., Schubert, W., Isom, P., Moslemy, P., *et al.* Trans-scleral iontophoretic delivery of low molecular weight therapeutics. *J Control Release* **147**(2), 225–231 (2010).

156. Patane, M.A., Schubert, W., Sanford, T., Gee, R., Burgos, M., Isom, W.P. *et al.* Evaluation of ocular and general safety following repeated dosing of dexamethasone phosphate delivered by transscleral iontophoresis in rabbits. *J Ocul Pharmacol Ther* **29**(8), 760–769 (2013).

157. Bar-Yehuda, S., Silverman, M.H., Kerns, W.D., Ochaion, A., Cohen, S., Fishman, P. The anti-inflammatory effect of A3 adenosine receptor agonists: A novel targeted therapy for rheumatoid arthritis. *Expert Opin Investig Drugs* **16**(10), 1601–1613 (2007).

158. Mabley, J., Soriano, F., Pacher, P., Hasko, G., Marton, A., Wallace, R., *et al.* The adenosine A3 receptor agonist, N6-(3-iodobenzyl)-adenosine-5'-N-methyluronamide, is protective in two murine models of colitis. *Eur J Pharm* **466**(3), 323–329 (2003).

159. Bar-Yehuda, S., Rath-Wolfson, L., Del Valle, L., Ochaion, A., Cohen, S., Patoka, R., *et al.* Induction of an antiinflammatory effect and prevention of cartilage damage in rat knee osteoarthritis by CF101 treatment. *Arthritis Rheum* **60**(10), 3061–3071 (2009).

160. Lee, H.T., Kim, M., Joo, J.D., Gallos, G., Chen, J.F., Emala, C.W. A3 adenosine receptor activation decreases mortality and renal and hepatic injury in murine septic peritonitis. *Am J Physiol Regul Integr Comp Physiol* **291**(4), R959–969 (2006).

161. Avni, I., Garzozi, H.J., Barequet, I.S., Segev, F., Varssano, D., Sartani, G., *et al.* Treatment of dry eye syndrome with orally administered CF101: data from a phase 2 clinical trial. *Ophthalmology* **117**(7), 1287–1293 (2010).

162. Trial of CF101 to Treat Patients With Dry Eye Disease. http://clinicaltrials.gov/ct2/show/NCT01235234?term=CF101&rank=7 [Accessed Dec 2013].

163. Meyer, D.M., Jesson, M.I., Li, X., Elrick, M.M., Funckes-Shippy, C.L., Warner, J.D., *et al.* Anti-inflammatory activity and neutrophil reductions mediated by the JAK1/JAK3 inhibitor, CP-690,550, in rat adjuvant-induced arthritis. *J Inflamm (Lond)* **7**, 41 (2010).

164. Ghoreschi, K., Laurence, A., O'Shea JJ. Janus kinases in immune cell signaling. *Immunol Rev* **228**(1), 273–287 (2009).

165. Sosne, G., Qiu, P., Ousler, G.W., 3rd, Dunn, S.P., Crockford D. Thymosin beta4: a potential novel dry eye therapy. *Ann N Y Acad Sci* **1270**, 45–50 (2012).

166. Xu, T.J., Wang, Q., Ma, X.W., Zhang, Z., Zhang, W., Xue, X.C., *et al.* A novel dimeric thymosin beta 4 with enhanced activities accelerates the rate of wound healing. *Drug Design Dev Ther* **7**, 1075–1088 (2013).

167. Sosne, G., Qiu, P., Kurpakus-Wheater M. Thymosin beta 4: A novel corneal wound healing and anti-inflammatory agent. *Clin Ophthalmol* **1**(3), 201–207 (2007).
168. Ho, J.H., Tseng, K.C., Ma, W.H., Chen, K.H., Lee, O.K., Su, Y. Thymosin beta-4 upregulates anti-oxidative enzymes and protects human *cornea* epithelial cells against oxidative damage. *Br J Ophthalmol* **92**(7), 992–997 (2008).
169. Sosne, G., Qiu, P., Christopherson, P.L., Wheater, M.K. Thymosin beta 4 suppression of corneal NFkappaB: a potential anti-inflammatory pathway. *Exp Eye Res* **84**(4), 663–669 (2007).
170. Regenerx receives clinical study report for phase 2 dry eye trial. Available from:http://phx.corporate-ir.net/pheonix.zhtml?c-144396&p-irol-newsArticle&ID-1706893&highlight.
171. RGN-259 significantly improves signs and symptoms of severe dry eye in phase 2 clinical trial. Available from: http://www.regenerx.com/wt/page/pr_1325770801 [Accessed Nov 30, 2013].
172. Anglade, E., Yatscoff, R., Foster, R., Grau, U. Next-generation calcineurin inhibitors for ophthalmic indications. *Expert Opin Investig Drugs* **16**(10), 1525–1540 (2007).
173. Figueroa, M.S., Ciancas, E., Orte, L. Long-term follow-up of tacrolimus treatment in immune posterior uveitis. *Eur J Ophthalmol* **17**(1), 69–74 (2007).
174. Hogan, A.C., McAvoy, C.E., Dick, A.D., Lee, R.W. Long-term efficacy and tolerance of tacrolimus for the treatment of uveitis. *Ophthalmology* **114**(5), 1000–1006 (2007).
175. Fei, W.L., Chen, J.Q., Yuan, J., Quan, D.P., Zhou, S.Y. Preliminary study of the effect of FK506 nanospheric-suspension eye drops on rejection of penetrating keratoplasty. *J Ocul Pharmacol Ther* **24**(2), 235–244 (2008).
176. Attas-Fox, L., Barkana, Y., Iskhakov, V., Rayvich, S., Gerber, Y., Morad, Y., *et al.* Topical tacrolimus 0.03% ointment for intractable allergic conjunctivitis: an open-label pilot study. *Curr Eye Res* **33**(7), 545–549 (2008).
177. Shoji, J., Sakimoto, T., Muromoto, K., Inada, N., Sawa, M., Ra, C. Comparison of topical dexamethasone and topical FK506 treatment for the experimental allergic conjunctivitis model in BALB/c mice. *Jpn J Ophthalmol* **49**(3), 205–210 (2005).
178. Fujita, E., Teramura, Y., Shiraga, T., Yoshioka, S., Iwatsubo, T., Kawamura, A., *et al.* Pharmacokinetics and tissue distribution of tacrolimus (FK506) after a single or repeated ocular instillation in rabbits. *J Ocul Pharmacol Ther* **24**(3), 309–319 (2008).
179. Moscovici, B.K., Holzchuh, R., Chiacchio, B.B., Santo, R.M., Shimazaki, J., Hida, R.Y. Clinical treatment of dry eye using 0.03% tacrolimus eye drops. *Cornea* **31**(8), 945–949 (2012).

180. Li, Z., Choi, W., Oh, H.J., Yoon, K.C. Effectiveness of topical infliximab in a mouse model of experimental dry eye. *Cornea* 31 Suppl 1, S25–31 (2012).

181. Dinarello, C.A. Interleukin-1 in the pathogenesis and treatment of inflammatory diseases. *Blood* 117(14), 3720–3732 (2011).

182. Le Loet, X., Nordstrom, D., Rodriguez, M., Rubbert, A., Sarzi-Puttini, P., Wouters, J.M., *et al.* Effect of anakinra on functional status in patients with active rheumatoid arthritis receiving concomitant therapy with traditional disease modifying antirheumatic drugs: evidence from the OMEGA Trial. *J Rheumatol* 35(8), 1538–1544 (2008).

183. Okanobo, A., Chauhan, S.K., Dastjerdi, M.H., Kodati, S., Dana, R. Efficacy of topical blockade of interleukin-1 in experimental dry eye disease. *Am J Ophthalmol* 154(1), 63–71 (2012).

184. Amparo, F., Dastjerdi, M.H., Okanobo, A., Ferrari, G., Smaga, L., Hamrah, P., *et al.* Topical interleukin 1 receptor antagonist for treatment of dry eye disease: a randomized clinical trial. *JAMA ophthalmology.* 131(6), 715–723 (2013).

185. Goldstein, M., Agahigian, J., Zarbis-Papstoitsis, G, Golden, K., *et al.* Use of Novel IL-1 Receptor Inhibitor (EBI-005) in the treatment of patietns with moderate to severe dry eye disease. Eleven Biotehrapeutics, Cambride MA. TFO.S., Friday, September 20, 2013, Poster Session II.

186. Lambiase, A., Manni, L., Bonini, S., Rama, P., Micera, A., Aloe, L. Nerve growth factor promotes corneal healing: structural, biochemical, and molecular analyses of rat and human corneas. *Invest Ophthalmol Vis Sci* 41(5), 1063–1069 (2000).

187. Joo, M.J., Yuhan, K.R., Hyon, J.Y., Lai, H., Hose, S., Sinha, D., *et al.* The effect of nerve growth factor on corneal sensitivity after laser in situ keratomileusis. *Arch Ophthalmol* 122(9), 1338–1341 (2004).

188. Esquenazi, S., Bazan, H.E., Bui, V., He, J., Kim, D.B., Bazan, N.G. Topical combination of NGF and DHA increases rabbit corneal nerve regeneration after photorefractive keratectomy. *Invest Ophthalmol Vis Sci* 46(9), 3121–3127 (2005).

189. Meerovitch, K., Torkildsen, G., Lonsdale, J., Goldfarb, H., Lama, T., Cumberlidge, G., *et al.* Safety and efficacy of MIM–D3 ophthalmic solutions in a randomized, placebo-controlled Phase 2 clinical trial in patients with dry eye. *Clin Ophthalmol* 7, 1275–1285 (2013).

Chapter 5: Ocular Inflammation Therapy

Seanna Grob,* Igor Kozak[†] and Kang Zhang[‡]

*Massachusetts Eye and Ear Infirmary,
Harvard Medical School, Boston, MA

[†]King Khaled Eye Specialist Hospital,
Riyadh, Saudi Arabia

[‡]Shiley Eye Institute, University of California San Diego,
La Jolla, CA

1. Introduction

Uveitis, or ocular inflammation, is a potentially blinding disease that comprises a wide array of diseases that affect the eyes. Vision threatening complications of this disease most commonly involve anterior chamber cellular reaction and cystoid macular edema, but also include band keratopathy, secondary glaucoma, secondary cataract, vitreous opacities, optic neuropathy, retinal scars and phthisis. Uveitis is the third leading cause of blindness with a prevalence of approximately 2.3 million people in the United States (US).[1] It has been estimated that 35% of patients with uveitis exhibit blindness or visual impairment.[2]

Uveitis is also a disease that predominately affects a younger, working class age group. Therefore, the economic costs of uveitis are predictably significant as visual impairment from uveitis affects persons in their most economically productive years.

Despite the economic and medical impact of this disease, relatively few randomized controlled trials have been performed for uveitis. However, the care and management of uveitis and ocular inflammatory disorders is poised to make evolutionary, if not revolutionary, changes in the years ahead. Our expanding understanding of the immune system has recently given rise to a diverse array of different targets, strategies and agents, especially for treatment of rheumatologic and autoimmune disease. The application of some of these medications in ocular disease has already taken place. In addition, the advancement in options for drug delivery systems has given rise to a number of new application devices and medicated devices that allow for long-term, targeted therapy for ocular inflammation.

In this chapter, we will discuss the current status of ocular drug therapies for ocular inflammation and inflammatory diseases, highlighting the newest innovations and ideas for drugs and drug delivery systems.

2. Ocular Inflammatory Diseases

Uveitis encompasses a very diverse array of diseases in etiology, location within the eye, and severity. Uveitis can range from an anterior uveitis managed with topical corticosteroids, or can involve sight-threatening diseases like Behçet's disease requiring aggressive systemic immunosuppression.

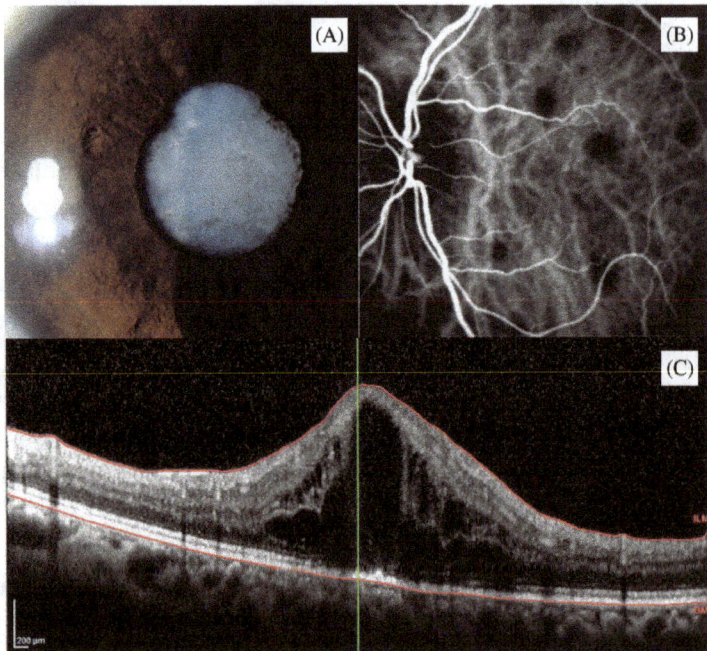

Figure 1.   Effects of intraocular inflammation on structures of the eye. (A) Complicated cataract due to uveitis. (B) Indocyanine green angiogram (ICG) showing multifocal choroiditis in Vogt-Koyanagi-Harada (VKH). (C) Macular edema in a patient with idiopathic uveitis.

The term "uveitis" describes any inflammation within the eye including the uvea, which comprises the iris, ciliary body and choroid as well as the sclera, retina, vitreous and optic nerve. Uveitis also describes infectious, non-infectious, and idiopathic conditions that can be localized to the eye or may also manifest systemically. Infectious etiologies include diseases such as toxoplasmosis, syphilis, bartonella, Lyme disease. Non-infectious etiologies often have an autoimmune component and include diseases such as sarcoidosis, Kawasaki's disease, systemic lupus erythematous, multiple sclerosis, and psoriasis. Uveitis can also be idiopathic and limited to the eye, as in birdshot retinochoroiditis. The current classification of uveitis was developed by the International Uveitis Study Group which based classification on anatomic location: anterior, intermediate, posterior, and panuveitis (Table 1).[3]

Table 1. Classification of uveitis.

Type of Uveitis	Anatomical Location	Noninfectious Systemic Diseases	Infectious Diseases
Anterior	Iritis Iridocyclitis Anterior cyclitis	Ankylosing spondylitis Behcet's syndrome Inflammatory bowel disease Juvenile idiopathic arthritis Sarcoidosis Seronegative arthropathy, Reiter syndrome	Herpes simplex virus Syphilis Tuberculosis Varicella zoster virus
Intermediate	Posterior cyclitis Pars planitis Hyalitis	Lymphoma Multiple sclerosis Sarcoidosis	Tuberculosis Lyme disease Syphilis
Posterior and Panuveitis	Retinitis Retinochorioditis Chorioretinitis Choroiditis Papilitis Diffuse uveitis, Endopthalmitis	Behcet's syndrome Lymphoma Sarcoidosis Vogt-Koyanagi-Harada syndrome	Cytomegalovirus Endogenous endopthalmitis Herpes simplex virus Syphilis Toxocariasis Toxoplasmosis Tuberculosis Varicella zoster virus

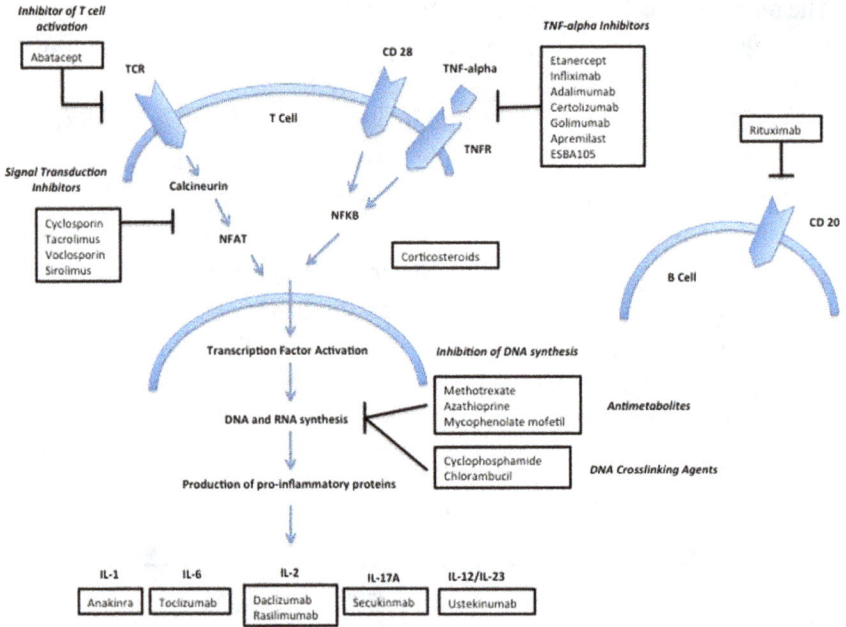

Figure 2. Inflammatory cascade and drug targets.

3. Inflammatory Casacade Overview

Inflammation is a product of a complex system of biologic structures and processes within the body. Years of research have provided details regarding all of the players involved in the inflammatory cascade and their specific targets. This information has allowed for advancements in drug discovery for treatment of inflammation and autoimmune diseases. Below is a brief overview of some of the drugs available and their associated inflammatory targets.

4. Ocular Drugs and Delivery Systems in Ocular Inflammation

4.1. *Nonsteroidal anti-inflammatory drugs*

Nonsteroidal anti-inflammatory drugs (NSAIDs) are one of the most widely available medications worldwide and have been increasingly

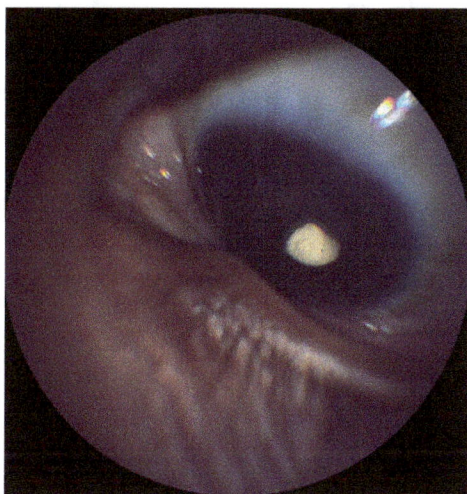

Figure 3.   Intraocular retisert implant.

employed in ophthalmology for the treatment of a wide range of ocular disorders. They are well-known medications that act by inhibiting cyclooxygenase and the production of prostaglandins that mediate inflammatory processes.

4.1.1. Topical non-steroidal anti-inflammatory drugs

There is good evidence for the use of topical NSAIDs for treatment of peri-operative anti-inflammatory effects, especially for cataract surgery.[4, 5] Randomized, prospective, double-masked, placebo, and active drug-controlled clinical studies with adequate numbers of patients have shown that topically applied 1% indomethacin, 0.03% flurbiprofen, 0.4% and 0.5% ketorolac, 0.1% diclofenac, 0.1% nepafenac, and 0.09% bromfenac all decrease postoperative inflammation after cataract surgery without significant toxicity when used as directed.[6] However, only diclofenac, ketorolac, nepafenac, and bromfenac are FDA-approved for this use, with the latter two being the newer NSAIDs on the market. Studies using topical NSAIDs have also shown evidence of a beneficial effect on visual acuity outcomes following cataract and retinal surgery. In addition, the use of topical NSAIDs has proven to be effective in decreasing ocular inflammation after strabismus[7,8] and vitreoretinal surgery,[9,10] with only a modest response after laser trabeculoplasty or cyclocryotherapy for treatment of glaucoma.[11–13]

Although NSAIDs have been of great use in the field of ophthalmology for the reduction of post-surgical inflammation, there is little clinical evidence supporting the use of NSAIDs in the treatment of uveitis. Two prospective, randomized studies involving patients with acute, nongranulomatous uveitis found higher cure rates among patients treated with 0.5% prednisolone disodium phosphate and 0.1% betamethasone disodium phosphate versus non-commercially available NSAID preparation, 5% tolmetin sodium dehydrate.[14,15] However, animal model studies have shown good aqueous penetration and equal efficacy to prednisolone acetate 1% in controlling uveitis (See Table 2).[16]

4.1.2. Systemic non-steroidal anti-inflammatory drugs

Systemic NSAIDs have also been discussed in the literature and have found therapeutic value in ocular disease. Oral and intravenous NSAIDs have been put to use in conditions such as orbital pseudotumor,[17,18] episcleritis,[19,20] and scleritis.[18] Systemic NSAIDs are used as first-line agents in scleritis with an overall response rate of 30–92% reported for diffuse and nodular anterior scleritis.[18] Indomethacine 25–50 mg three times a day is the most commonly utilized treatment regimen. These medications should be taken with an H_2-blocker or a proton-pump inhibitor to prevent gastric upset or ulcer formation.

4.2. *Glucocorticosteroids*

Corticosteroids remain the mainstay therapy of ocular inflammation. Their use is quite common among ophthalmologists, especially for the treatment of ocular inflammatory disorders. Steroids are both anti-inflammatory and immunosuppressive. Corticosteroids bind intracellular receptors that translocate into the nucleus, where the drug is involved in altering DNA transcription into mRNA. Ultimately, these alterations in DNA transcription prevent the synthesis and release of inflammatory mediators

Table 2. Non-steroidal anti-inflammatory drugs.

Drug	Administration	Manufacturer	Indication
Bromfenac 0.09% solution (Bromday®)	Topical	Ista	*Post-operative inflammation and ocular pain after cataract extraction
Diclofenac 0.1% solution (Voltaren®)	Topical	generic	*Post-operative inflammation and ocular pain after cataract extraction *Relief of pain and photophobia in patient undergoing corneal refractive surgery
Flurbiprofen sodium 0.03% solution (Ocufen®)	Topical	generic	*Inhibition of intraoperative miosis
Ketorolac tromethamine 0.5% solution (Acular®)	Topical	Allergan	*Relief of ocular itching related to seasonal allergic conjunctivitis *Post-operative inflammation and ocular pain after cataract extraction
Ketorolac tromethamine 0.4% solution (Acular LS®)	Topical	Allergan	*Post-operative inflammation and ocular pain after cataract extraction
Nepafenac 0.1% suspension (Nevanac™)	Topical	Alcon	*Post-operative inflammation and ocular pain after cataract extraction
Indomethacine 0.1% solution	Topical	Bausch + Lomb	*Post-operative inflammation and ocular pain after cataract extraction
Indomethacine	Systemic	generic	*Treatment of ocular pain and inflammation from scleritis, episcleritis, pseudotumor

and the recruitment of T lymphocytes and other effector cells into sites of inflammation.

Steroids can be used in a targeted, local fashion (topical, peri-bulbar, intravitreal) or they can be used systemically (oral or intravenous steroids). The benefits of local therapy are a decrease in the risk of systemic side effects associated with steroid use. With the exception of a new agent, difluprednate, most of the advances in steroid therapy entail novel delivery systems providing options for extended release therapy. Below we will discuss the different delivery systems of corticosteroids, their uses and benefits in the treatment of ocular inflammation, and their potential complications.

4.2.1. Topical corticosteroids

Topical steroids are a part of the standard practice in the treatment of anterior uveitis and post-surgical inflammation. The goal of therapy is to rapidly decrease the intraocular inflammation in order to prevent ocular damage, scarring, and ultimately vision loss. These medications can be dosed as often as every 30 minutes for severe inflammatory reactions (Table 3).

While these agents are very effective in treating ocular inflammation, they are not without associated risks. The ocular side effects of steroid use for all types and means of administration include cataract formation and increased intraocular pressure. These side effects are related to the strength of the particular steroid and their ocular penetration.[21] The most potent steroids, prednisolone acetate and B-methasone, are notorious for their side effects. The potency of systemic steroids is based on their ability to bind the intracellular receptor, whereas the potency of topical steroid is more related to corneal penetration and intraocular metabolism. Studies using techniques such as anterior chamber fluorophotometry have suggested that dexamethasone sodium 0.1% and prednisolone acetate 1% are broadly equivalent.[22,23]

Rimexolone is a topical corticosteroid specifically engineered by eliminating a hydroxyl group to generate less effect on intraocular pressure. Randomized controlled trials suggest less of an intraocular pressure rise

Table 3. Topical ophthalmic corticosteroids.

Brand name	Generic name	Manufacturer	Approved Dosing
Alrex®	loteprednol 0.2%	Bausch + Lomb	q.i.d.
Durezol®	difluprenate 0.05%	Alcon	q.i.d. for 2 weeks, then b.i.d. for 1 week, and then gradual taper
FML®	fluorometholone alcohol 0.1%	Allergan	Up to q4h for first 24 to 48 hrs; or b.i.d. to q.i.d., then gradual taper
Lotemax®	loteprednol 0.5%	Bausch + Lomb	Up to qh for first week; or q.i.d. for 2 weeks, then gradual taper
Pred Forte®	prednisolone acetate 1%	Allergan	Up to q.i.d. for first 24 to 48 hrs; or b.i.d. to q.i.d., then gradual taper
N/A	prednisolone sodium phosphate 1%	generic	Up to qh during the day, q2h during the night as initial therapy; or q4h, then t.i.d. to q.i.d, then gradual taper

with Rimexolone as compared to either dexamethasone sodium 0.1% and prednisolone acetate 1%.[24,25] However, studies suggest no significant difference in effectiveness controlling intraocular inflammation in acute anterior uveitis.[24] Therefore, this medication may benefit patients with known glaucoma or significant response to corticosteroid use. Letoprednol etabonate 0.5% is also associated with less of an intraocular pressure rise, but it has poorer eye penetrance and therefore would best be used for surface inflammation.[25]

Difluprednate is a novel prednisolone derivative approved on June 24, 2008 by the US Food and Drug Administration (FDA) for the treatment of postoperative inflammation and pain. Difluprednate ophthalmic solution 0.05% (Durezol®) was developed and marketed by Sirion Therapeutics, Inc. Alcon Laboratories (Fort Worth, TX) has since licensed Durezol® from Sirion Therapeutics, Inc. Difluprednate has a high glucocorticoid receptor binding affinity due to fluorination at the C-6 and C-9 positions, superior tissue penetration as a result of the addition of butyrate and acetate esters at positions C-17 and C-21,[26,27] and its increased bioavailability due to its formulation as an emulsion rather than a suspension.

Randomized, double-masked, placebo-controlled clinical trials involving 26 clinics in the US have established effectiveness and safety of topical difluprednate ophthalmic solution 0.05% dosed at one drop two times a day (b.i.d) or one drop four times a day (q.i.d) for 14 days followed by a 2 week taper period for the treatment of inflammation and pain associated with ocular surgery.[28] Clinical response, defined as anterior chamber cell count less than 5 and flare grade 0, was noted as early as 3 days post-operatively. In addition, by day 29, 87 of 110 and 88 of 107 patients in the difluprednate b.i.d and q.i.d groups achieved clinical response as compared to 59 of the 218 patients in the placebo group.

Currently difluprednate ophthalmic emulsion is being studied for the use of other ocular inflammatory diseases, including a US Phase III study evaluating difluprednate for the treatment of anterior uveitis. This Phase III, randomized trial involving 22 clinics in the US established the effectiveness and safety of difluprednate 0.05% emulsion when compared to prednisolone acetate 1% suspension.[29] A non-inferiority study, compared difluprednate q.i.d to prednisolone eight times a day, and not only found anterior chamber cell grade improvement to be at least equivalent between the two treatment regimens, but also found best corrected visual acuity (BCVA) to be better and the number of patients who failed treatment to be less in the difluprednate group. Due to the less frequent dosing regimen, it would be reasonable to assume difluprednate would be associated with better treatment compliance as a treatment regimen compared to prednisolone every 30 minutes, which is more at risk for missing important drops. In addition, evaluation of safety profiles showed increase in intraocular pressure (IOP) to be similar between the two groups.

4.2.2. Systemic corticosteroids

Systemic corticosteroids are generally advocated for intermediate and posterior uveitis, especially when the case involves bilateral or systemic disease.[30–32] The ocular penetration of systemic steroids is significant, even in eyes with an intact blood-retinal barrier.[33,34] Radiographic localization has demonstrated that systemically administered dexamethasone is able to penetrate cells in the choroid, retina, and sclera better than topical application.[35]

When deciding between oral and intravenous (IV) steroids, oral steroids are often preferred because of their ease of use and lack of requirement for hospital admission. The dosage of oral steroids depends on disease severity, previous response to treatment, presence of associated systemic disease as well as age and weight in children.[31] Typically, the adult starting dose is 1–2 mg of prednisolone per kilogram per day until the inflammation is under control and then the dosing is slowly tapered. The goal is to achieve inflammatory control at a dose of 7.5 mg or less, and if this cannot be achieved, an adjunctive therapy needs to be considered. The side effects of oral steroids are numerous including gastric ulcers, diabetes, hypertension, weight gain, psychological disturbances, and growth suppression in children.[36] Therefore, close monitoring of the patients blood pressure, blood sugar, height and weight, and development of osteopenia or osteoporosis is important.

Intravenous high dose steroids may achieve necessary concentrations for treatment, but these benefits are often outweighed by the systemic side effects associated with IV corticosteroids. IV corticosteroids should be reserved for severe sight-threatening cases of uveitis where rapid control of inflammation is vital. Treatment with IV corticosteroids has shown to be effective in the treatment of Behçet's disease, Vogt-Koyanagi-Harada (VKH) syndrome, serpiginous choroiditis and uveitis associated with multiple sclerosis.[37–40] IV methylprednisone is dosed at 1 mg/kg/day and then tapered after disease severity improves. Hospitalization is required not only for IV administration, but also for close monitoring of potential severe side effects, including seizures, anaphylactic reactions, and sudden death; however these severe reactions are rare.[37]

4.2.3. Periocular corticosteroids

The major limitation to topical corticosteroid therapy is its inability to reach necessary concentrations to effectively treat posterior uveitis.

Periocular or intraocular injections, therefore, are a useful alternative. Periocular corticosteroid administration is best utilized in patients with unilateral or asymmetric disease, or in patients in whom systemic steroids are less desirable, e.g. pregnant patients, or patients with history of adverse reaction to systemic steroids. Periocular corticosteroid injections can be administered either via the sub-Tenon route or as an orbital floor injection. Both of these injection methods are safe, with low risk of ocular penetration and developing other side effects, such as increased IOP and/or cataract.[41–44]

Periocular injections successfully reach an appropriate concentration to control ocular inflammation;[41–44] however, the mechanisms of entrance into the eye is unknown.[32] A significant benefit is that local levels of the drug remain, even after 30 days,[45] while systemic levels of the drug are low. The use of transcleral enhancers may in the future increase intravitreal concentration of corticosteroids after periocular administration.[46] Therefore, systemic side effects can also be avoided with this method.

4.2.4. Intravitreal injections of corticosteroids

Intravitreal injections of triamcinolone acetonide (IVTA) is most commonly used in the treatment of posterior uveitis and inflammatory cystoid macular edema (CME). It involves injection of corticosteroid directly into the vitreous body, thus allowing for a higher concentration of intraocular corticosteroid[47] with a decreased risk of systemic side effects. The dose often used is 4 mg, with the typical duration of effect lasting 4–5 months. High dose triamcinolone acetonide has also been used in clinical practice.[48,49]

CME is one of the most common causes of visual loss in patients with uveitis.[2,50] Vision loss is due to the photoreceptor cell damage from untreated or poorly controlled CME. A study examining the use of IVTA in patients with quiescent uveitis found resolution of CME in 29% of 24 eyes in patients with up to three injections and a significant decrease in retinal thickness; while visual acuity improved greater than two lines in 37.5% of patients up to 12 weeks after the first injection.[50] IVTA has been shown to be somewhat more effective in younger patients. IVTA has also been shown to be effective in treating uveitis caused by systemic diseases such as Behçet's disease,[51,52] sympathetic ophthalmia,[53,54] and VKH.[55]

Although serum levels of corticosteroid are not significant after IVTA, these injections are not without local risk factors. Raised IOP is seen in 29–50% of patients within a year. Often, the increased IOP can be managed medically with tropical drops. However, a few patients end up needing filtration surgery to control IOP elevation. Cataract formation is also a common finding in patients who have had IVTA injections and the rate of cataract progression is reported to be 5-fold. Other side effects includes endophthalmitis, intravitreal hemorrhage, rhegmatogenous retinal detachment, and central retinal vein occlusion; however, these risks are rare.

4.2.5. Intravitreal implants

Other methods of corticosteroid delivery systems to the eye have been explored. These novel methods provide a means for local, targeted drug delivery over a sustained period of time, from days to months. The benefits of these implants include long-term control of intraocular inflammation leading to a decrease in the number of relapses of intraocular inflammation, and therefore the potential for less ocular damage.

4.2.5.1. Retisert® implant

The fluocinolone acetonide implant (Retisert; Bausch & Lomb, Rochester, New York, NY) is a non-biodegradable sustained delivery corticosteroid. This implant has been approved by the FDA for use in patients with severe posterior uveitis. Each implant consists of a siliocone elastomer containing fluocinolone acetonide 0.59 mg. It delivers the drug at an initial rate of 0.6 µg/day over the first month, decreasing to a steady rate of 0.3–0.4 µg/day over approximately 30 months. Fluocinolone acetonide was chosen for its high potency, low solubility, and very short action in the systemic circulation — allowing for a small steroid pellet and a lower risk of systemic side effects. Pharmacokinetic studies in rabbits have demonstrated the delivery of constant levels of corticosteroid to the posterior pole with no evidence of systemic absorption.[56,57]

Implantation involves surgical placement of the implant in the vitreous cavity and is a procedure that most retinal specialists can easily master. Complications related to placement of the implant can include suprachoroidal placement, issues with wound healing, scleral thinning over the implant, or infection.

Small preliminary studies in patients with non-infections posterior uveitis demonstrated the efficacy of the Retisert® implant in controlling ocular inflammation. The efficacy has since been confirmed in a larger study with 278 patients. The Multicenter Uveitis Steroid Treatment Trial is a study aimed to determine whether control of intermediate or posterior uveitis with Retisert® implants achieves the same or better visual acuity at 2 years when compared to oral systemic therapy.[58] Results from the 24-month analysis showed mean visual acuity improvement over 24 months, with neither approach being superior. However, residual active uveitis was higher in the systemically treated group ($p = 0.001$).[59]

The fluocinolone acetonide implant has been strongly associated with the development of cataracts, with over 93% of phakic patients undergoing cataract surgery during the 3-year post-implantation period.[60] It is also associated with a high rate of IOP rise. Studies report up to 10 mmHg increase in mean IOP over 60–70% of patients that require an average of 3.3 IOP lowering medications and over 30–40% of patients require glaucoma surgery following implant insertion.[60–63] When comparing Retisert® to systemic therapy, Retisert® was found to have a higher risk of cataract surgery and glaucoma, whereas systemic therapy was more associated with prescription-requiring infections.[59] Therefore, patients should be appropriately educated about the higher likelihood of requiring cataract and glaucoma surgery.

4.2.5.2. Ozurdex®

The Dexamethasone Posterior Segment Drug Delivery System® (Dexamethasone DDS; Allergan, Inc., Irvine, CA) is a biodegradable implant that is injected into the vitreous and gradually releases dexamethasone over the course of 6 months after insertion. The implant utilizes a

Novadur™ solid polymer delivery system, in which biodegradable material is combined with dexamethasone to form a small rod-shaped implant that can now be injected with a specially designed injector in an office-setting. The implant was approved by the FDA in 2009 for the treatment of macular edema in patients following branch or central retinal vein occlusion and is now marketed as Ozurdex®.[64]

In the first Phase II clinical trials, implants with two different doses of 350 µg and 700 µg of dexamtheasone were compared to sham in patients with CME, from a number of causes. BCVA improved by 10 letters or more in 35% of patients with the higher-dose implant and 24% of those with the lower dose implant and 13% of the sham-treated patients by day 90.[65,66] Phase III clinical studies have shown that patients receiving the dexamethaxone implants when compared to sham achieved a 15-letter improvement in BCVA much faster than eyes receiving the sham treatment. A subgroup analysis also found that response to the implant was often greater in eyes known to have a shorter duration of macular edema.[64]

Recent clinical studies have evaluated the safety and efficacy of the dexamethasone implant as monotherapy for uveitic and diabetic macular edema. In addition, the dexamethosone implant has been investigated for use in vitrectomized patients, in a combination therapy of laser photocoagulation in diabetic macular edema, as well as in combination with ranimizumab (Lucentis, Genentech, Inc, San Francisco, CA) in patients with choroidal neovascularization (CNV) secondary to exudative age-related macular degeneration. The findings of these studies indicate that dexamethasone implants improve visual acuity and intraocular inflammation in uveitic macular edema patients and in difficult-to-treat vitrectomized patients, and reduces the need for repeated ranibizumab injections in patients with CNV.

One significant benefit is that the implant is placed using an office-based procedure and the patient then avoids a trip to the operating room. In addition, there is a lower risk for the development of elevated IOP and cataract. Compared to the fluocinolone acetonide implant, only 17% of patients in the 700-µg dose of dexamethasone DDS group developed an IOP increase of 10-mmHg or more from baseline.[65]

4.2.5.3. Other implants

Iluvien (Alimera Sciences Inc., Alpharetta, GA, USA) is a fluocinolone acetonide intravitreal insert that delivers a low dose (0.2 or 0.5 μg/day) of corticosteroid for up to 3 years. It utilizes the same drug matrix as Retisert®, but has lower dosage of steroid and is another implant that can be injected in an outpatient setting. After the medication is depleted, the insert is designed to remain in the eye.

The Fluocinolone Acetonide in Diabetic Macular Edema (FAME) study consists of two 3-year Phase III masked, randomized, multi-center trials with 956 patients in the US, Canada, Europe, and India that assesses the safety and efficacy of Iluvien® in the treatment of Diabetic Macular Edema. The three treatment arms consist of high dose Iluvien®, low dose Iluvien® and control. The primary end point for efficacy of this therapy was the difference in the percentage of the patients whose BCVA improved by 15 or more letters from baseline on the Early Treatment Diabetic Retinopathy Study (ETDRS) eye chart at 24 months. The combined data from both trials has shown statistically significant effects maintained through 36 months.[67]

The I-vation™ implant (SurModics Inc.) uses triamcinolone acetonide and has been reported to have a duration of over one year. The mechanism of implantation involves a screw-shaped device that is twisted through the pars plana. Phase I clinical trials were designed to evaluate the safety, tolerability, and efficacy of this implant for the treatment of DME (Table 4).[68]

4.3. Immunomodulatory therapy

Corticosteroids are an essential modality in treating ocular inflammation; however, their potential side effects are notorious and damaging in the long term. Although the use of steroids is often essential in the treatment of acute inflammation, the goal is to control the acute inflammatory reaction and then use steroid-sparing therapies to keep the disease in remission. Steroid sparing immunomodulatory therapy (IMT) may be accomplished using chemotherapeutic agents, biologic response modifiers, or a combination of the two.

Table 4. Intravitreal steroid implants.

Implant	Manufacturer	Corticosteroid	Mechanism of Administration	Potential or Approved Uses
Retisert®	Bausch + Lomb	Fluocinolone acetonide	Surgical implantation into the vitreous cavity	*Proposed treatment for control of intermediate or posterior uveitis
Ozurdex®	Allergan	Dexamethasone	Injected into vitreous cavity in office-setting	*FDA-approved for treatment of macular edema following branch or central retinal vein occlusion
Iluvien®	Alimera Sciences Inc.	Fluocinolone acetonide	Injected into vitreous cavity in office-setting	*Proposed reatment of diabetic macular edema
I-vation™	SurModics Inc.	Triamcinolone acetonide	Screw-shaped device twisted through pars plana	*Proposed treatment of diabetic macular edema

The Systemic Immunosuppresive Therapy for Diseases (SITE) retrospective cohort studies have contributed information regarding the efficacy and safety of multiple IMTs in the treatment of ocular inflammatory disorders. Its main objective was to determine if IMT is associated with an increase in the prevalence of cancer when compared to the general population. Below we will discuss a variety of agents that have been studied for the treatment of ocular inflammation and will include data from SITE and other relevant clinical trials.

4.3.1. Chemotherapeutic agents

4.3.1.1. Antimetabolites

Antimetabolites are immunosuppressive agents that primarily function in the disruption of DNA synthesis. They have been available for over 50 years and are most commonly used in treating rheumatologic and autoimmune diseases.

4.3.1.1.1. Methotrexate

Methotrexate is a disease modifying anti-rheumatic drug (DMARD) which inhibits DNA synthesis by acting as a folate analog and inactivates the enzyme dihydrofolate reductase (DHFR). DHFR converts dihydrofolate to tetrahydrofolate, a methyl group shuttle required for the synthesis of purines, thymidylic acid, and certain amino acids. The therapeutic effect of low-dose methotrexate may be explained by its anti-angiogenic properties, its inhibition of cytokine production, cellular and humoral immunosuppression, and its inhibition of DHFR and other folate-dependent enzymes.

Methotrexate is available in oral, subcutaneous, and intravenous forms. It is given in doses of 7.5 mg up to 50 mg once a week. A total of 3–6 weeks are required for methotrexate to take effect.

SITE evaluated 384 patients with multiple different ocular inflammatory diseases treated with methotrexate as the sole non-corticosteroid immunosuppressant agent. Methotrexate was found to achieve quiescence of ocular inflammation in 66% of patients within 1 year, which allowed for successful tapering of systemic corticosteroids to 10 mg/day or less in

58% of patients. Treatment success was the most common in patients with anterior uveitis and scleritis with inflammatory control at approximately 56% in both diseases. However, there was a high rate, 42%, of patient-initiated discontinuation of the medication either from ineffectiveness or side effects.[69]

The most concerning side effect related to methotrexate is the increased risk of malignancy. However, SITE showed no increased risk of mortality or malignancy in patients treated with methotrexate when compared to controls.[70] The most common side effects are ulcerative stomatitis, gastrointestinal upset, fatigue, transaminitis, and low white blood cell count. The Massachusetts Eye Research and Surgery Institution (MERSI) recommend the screening of complete blood count (CBC), liver function tests (LFTs) and creatinine at 6 weeks intervals and folic acid supplementation 1 mg/day to prevent problems associated with folate deficiency.[71]

4.3.1.1.2. Azathioprine

Azathioprine is a prodrug for 6-mercaptopurine that mimics the purine structure and can act as a precursor to adenine and guanine synthesis, therefore interfering with DNA, RNA and ultimately protein synthesis. However, its immunosuppressive effects are also attributed to selective inhibition of T-lymphocyte function, suppression of homing in circulating T cells, selective reduction of monocyte precursors and the participation of NK cells in antibody-dependent cytotoxicity reactions, and the suppression of delayed Type IV hypersensitivity reaction in renal, skin, and cardiac allografts.

Studies have shown azathioprine to be effective in treating juvenile idiopathic arthritis (JIA) and intermediate and chronic uveitis.[70,72,73] In the SITE retrospective cohort study, 145 patients were treated with azathioprine for a number of different non-infectious ocular inflammatory diseases. The drug was found to control inflammation in 62% of patients with a steroid-sparing effect in 47% of patients in 1 year.

Azathioprine is typically prescribed with an initial dosage of 2–3 mg/kg/day orally and then adjustments are made depending on clinical response and side effects. The MERSI recommends an initial CBC with differential and liver function tests before beginning therapy and then at 4-week intervals for the duration of treatment to monitor for myelo-suppression and change in liver function. Other recommendations include weekly complete hemograms until disease activity, drug dosage, and hematologic parameters are stabilized and checking activity level of the enzyme thiopurine methyltransferase (TPMT) which is involved in the metabolism of azathioprine.[67] The goal of treatment is achieving lasting remission following cessation of therapy with no need for corticosteroid use.

4.3.1.1.3. Mycophenolate Mofetil

Mycophenolate Mofetil (MMF) (CellCept®, Roche, San Francisco, CA) is a prodrug and an inosine monophosphate dehydrogenase inhibitor that disrupts the *de novo* pathway of purine synthesis that is preferentially used by B and T cells in DNA synthesis. MMF also suppresses antibody synthesis, disrupts cell adhesion to vascular endothelium, and interferes with lymphocytic chemotaxis.

MMF is effective in treating uveitis either as monotherapy or in combination with steroids, methotrexate, azathioprine, and cyclosporine.[74] It can be used as a steroid-sparing agent or in patients unable to tolerate methotrexate. In the SITE cohort, control of ocular inflammation was achieved in 73% of the 236 patients treated with MMF.[75]

It is often prescribed as 1 g twice a day on an empty stomach. Dosages greater than 3 g/day have the potential of causing toxicity. Side effects are similar to the other antimetabolites discussed above and include gastrointestinal upset and myelosuppression. Therefore, complete blood cell count and liver function tests should be monitored every six weeks for changes.

The newer formulation of MMF is mycophenolic acid (Myfortic®, Novartis, East Hanover, NJ) and has been shown to cause less gastrointestinal side effects. The salt mycophenolate sodium has also been introduced.

4.3.1.2. Alkylating agents

Alkylating agents interfere with DNA replication by cross-linking nucleic acids, ultimately causing abnormal base pairing, failure of DNA replication, and termination of the cell cycle. They are most commonly used in the treatment of cancer and autoimmune diseases.

4.3.1.2.1. Cyclophosphamide

Cyclophosphamide is a nitrogen mustard alkylating agent that forms DNA crosslinks between and within DNA strands at guanine N-7 positions. The immunosuppressant effects are due to cytotoxicity of immunocompetent lymphocytes undergoing cell division.

Cyclophosphamide was first described in the treatment of steroid-resistant uveitis in 1952.[76] Since this time, cyclophosphamide has been shown to be effective in treating uveitis associated with systemic diseases such as Wegener's granulomatosis, rheumatoid arthritis, polyarteritis nodosa, and relapsing polychondritis.[77–80] As an adjunct agent, it has been shown to be more effective in combination with steroids when compared to steroids alone.[81] Uveitis can be treated with oral or pulsed IV therapy for short periods of time. Daily oral dosing includes 1–3 mg/kg/day of cyclophosphamide.

Common adverse drug reactions include low white blood cell count, hemorrhagic cystitis, teratogenicity and gastrointestinal upset. Of the 215 patients receiving cyclophosphamide therapy for inflammatory eye disease in the SITE cohort study, 18.1% had low white cell count and 7.7% had blood in the urine or cystitis.[69,82] Therefore, careful monitoring of the white cell count is necessary in order to avoid a patient's susceptibility to life threatening opportunistic infections. In addition, cyclophosphamide in itself is thought to be carcinogenic and the SITE study showed a possible increased risk of cancer mortality with this medication.[69]

4.3.1.2.2. Chlorambucil

Chlorambucil is also a nitrogen mustard alkylating agent that has an action similar to that of cyclophosphamide and ultimately interferes with DNA replication. At this time there are two treatment modalities. Chlorambucil can be given in low doses over the course of a year in an attempt to provide long-term remission. The other option includes high-dose, short-term therapy over 3–6 months with gradual increase in dosages each week until control of uveitis is attained.

Chlorambucil has not been as extensively studied as cyclophosphamide, but it has shown effectiveness in treating Behçet's disease, and intractable noninfectious uveitis associated with juvenile rheumatoid arthritis, pars planitis, sympathetic ophthalmia, Crohn's disease, and HLA-B27 associated uveitis. Studies associated with treatment of Behcet's disease showed that high-dose, short-term therapy is effective in preventing recurrence after 6–24 months of use.[83]

The potential side effects are similar to cyclophosphamide and therefore careful monitoring of the CBC is necessary.

4.3.1.3. Signal transduction inhibitors

4.3.1.3.1. Cyclosporine

Cyclosporine is an immunosuppressive agent derived from a fungus that binds to an intracellular protein, cyclophilin, which prevents the activation of calcineurin. Calcineurin is a calcium- and calmodulin-dependent phosphatase that activates nuclear factor of the activated T-cell (NFAT). NFAT then activates IL-2 and other cytokines that act on T-helper cell response. When cyclosporine inhibits the activation of calcineurin, NFAT cannot translocate into the nucleus of the cell and cannot provide the signal for the production of IL-2. The final effect is prevention of T lymphocyte activation.

Cyclosporine has demonstrated efficacy in the treatment of uveitis associated with Behçet's disease, sarcoidosis, and VKH syndrome. It reduces inflammation comparable to that of steroids when used as a monotherapy, but is often used in combination with steroids or other immunomodulating therapies. Cyclosporin is administered systemically for the treatment of uveitis and is taken in doses of 2–5 mg/kg per day. There is also a topical form of cyclosporine used in ophthalmology for the treatment of dry eyes (Restasis®, Allergan), but this should not be confused with the systemic medication for uveitis.

Side effects include nephrotoxicity, hypertension, hepatotoxicity, hypertrichosis, neuropathy, gingival hypertrophy, and GI upset. Therefore, it is important to regularly monitor a patient's vital signs and blood chemistries.

4.3.1.3.2. Tacrolimus

Tacrolimus is a macrolide antibiotic derivative of the bacterium *Streptomyces tsukubaensis* that is also involved in calcineurin inhibition. Tacrolimus binds to FK-506 binding protein 12 (FKBP12) to create a complex that interferes with the activity of calcineurin phosphatase, thereby affecting the same NFAT pathway as cyclosporin.

Tacrolimus is well known for its use in prevention of graft rejection. However, it is still an emerging therapy for uveitis in that it has not been as closely scrutinized as cyclosporin. However, it has been shown to be effective in one study in reducing inflammation that was refractory to cyclosporine therapy.[84] When comparing tacrolimus to cyclosporine, they demonstrated comparable efficacy and there was actually a lower incidence of hypertension and lipid abnormalities in the tacrolimus-treated patients.[85] Tacrolimus has also shown efficacy in providing steroid sparing effects, as patients have been able to taper their oral prednisone to less than 10 mg/day after 14 months of immune modulation monotherapy for uveitis.[86]

Tacrolimus is effective for treating uveitis in doses of 0.05 mg/kg/day. The potential side effects are similar to that of cyclosporine and therefore, blood pressure and kidney function need to be monitored. However, given the possible favorable side effect profile, some have advocated for use of tacrolimus instead of cyclosporine.[86]

4.3.1.3.3. Voclosporin

Voclosporin or Leveniq (Lux Biosciences, Jersey City, NJ) is a novel calcineurin inhibitor developed by modifying the functional group on cyclosporine. It was created with the intention of providing a therapy that is four times more potent than other calcineurin inhibitors. Voclosporin is dosed at 0.4 mg/kg orally twice a day. It was evaluated in a non-infectious uveitis trial, LUMINATE (Lux Uveitis Multicenter Investigation of a New

Approach to Treatment). Three randomized, double-blind, placebo-controlled, Phase II/III trials including patients with noninfectious, sight-threatening uveitis were performed. Results showed a superiority of voclosporin to placebo for the clearance of vitreous haze and a 50% decrease in recurrence rate of inflammation at 6 months with favorable side effect profiles in patients with intermediate, posterior, and panuveitis.[87] In all three clinical trials, 96–68% of patients were able to reduce their oral prednisone dosage to ≤ 5 mg daily. Future studies will be needed to confirm these results and provide data on clinical efficacy and a more favorable side effect profile.[88]

4.3.1.3.4. Sirolimus

Sirolimus, also known as rapamycin, is a macrolide antibiotic derived from *Streptomyces hydroscoious* that has a long history of use in cardiology and solid organ transplant; however, its use in ophthalmology is just now emerging. Sirolimus ultimately inhibits the cell cycle and proliferation of T lymphocytes by binding to FKBP-12 and inhibiting the mTOR pathway and activation of p70 kinase. In addition, the mTOR inhibition blunts the IL-2 receptor and CD28-dependent signaling pathways as well as blocks growth factor proliferation signaling and activation of HIF1-a, a potent activator of VEGF signaling. Given the number of different effects of sirolimus, it has become an intriguing prospect for use in a number of ophthalmic disease processes.

Sirolimus has been studied at systemic doses for the treatment of refractory uveitis and for uveitis-induced choroidal neovascular membranes.[89] It has also been evaluated for as an adjunct to anti-VEGF therapy for exudative age-related macular degeneration (AMD).[90] The systemic dosage is usually 2 mg/day in uveitis. Given the potential prospects of its use in ophthalmology, other modalities of administration have been developed. A local periocular/intravitreal formulation (Perceiva by MacuSight, now made by Santen) was created to provide local therapy without the risk of systemic side effects. Multiple clinical trials are now evaluating the safety and efficacy of this medication and the different formulations for the treatment of ocular inflammation. Clinical trials including Intravitreal Sirolimus as a Therapeutic Approach to Uveitis (SAVE [NCT00908466] and SAVE-2 [NCT01280669]) and Subconjunctival Sirolimus for Treatment of Autoimmune Active Anterior Uveitis (NCT00876434) are currently underway. Interestingly, subconjunctival injections have shown some superior efficacy when compared to intravitreal injections. This response is likely related to its lipophilic nature and ability for transcleral delivery. Further studies will confirm the safety and efficacy of the different formulations (See Table 5).

4.3.2. Biologic response modifiers

Biologic response modifiers (BRMs) is a term applied broadly to a group of drugs that target cytokines or signaling pathways. They have been revolutionary in the treatment of inflammatory disease and hold much promise in the treatment of uveitis in the future.

4.3.2.1. TNF-a inhibitors

Tumor necrosis factor- alpha (TNF-α) is a prominent target for therapy in immunological diseases. At least five drugs that target TNF-α are approved for the treatment of rheumatologic disease. The two broad strategies used in targeting TNF include a soluble receptor (etanercept) versus a targeting antibody (infliximab, adalimumab, certolizumab, golimumab). Their use in uveitis is steadily expanding.

Etanercept is unique in that most BRMs are monoclonal antibodies, whereas etanercept is a soluble, bivalent receptor for TNF-α. It competitively binds TNF-α, inactivating immune activities that rely on this factor for signal transduction. Etanercept has been effective in the treatment of arthritis, but its success in treatment of uveitis is conflicting.[67,91] Moreover, occasional worsening of uveitis has been noted.[92]

The other TNF-α inhibitors can be differentiated on their mode of delivery and the structure of the antibody. Infliximab or remicade® is the only chimeric and intravenous solution on the market. Its antigen-binding (Fab) domain is mouse while its Fc domain is human. Infliximab also has the largest amount of data amongst the other TNF-α inhibitors in its effectiveness and use in the treatment of ocular inflammatory disease. There have been studies demonstrating its effectiveness in treating refractory

Table 5. Chemotheapeutic agents.

Class	Drugs	Mechanism of Action	Ongoing Clinical Trials Identifier
Antimetabolites	Methotrexate	*Inhibits dihydrofolate reductase involved in DNA synthesis *Inhibits cytokine production *Cellular and humoral immunosuppresion	NCT01829295 NCT01232920
	Azathioprine	*Interferes with DNA synthesis *Selectively inhibits T-lymphocyte function *Suppresses homing in circulating T cells *Reduces monocyte precursors and the participation of NK cells in antibody-dependent cytotoxicity reactions *Suppresses delayed Type IV hypersensitivity reaction	
	Mycophenolate Mofetil	*Disrupts the de novo pathway of purine synthesis used by B and T cells in DNA synthesis *Suppresses antibody synthesis *Disrupts cell adhesion to vascular endothelium and interferes with lymphocytic chemotaxis	NCT01092533 NCT01232920 NCT01829295
Alkylating Agents	Cyclophosphamide	*Forms DNA cross-links and interferes with DNA replication *Cytotoxicity of immunocompetent lymphocytes undergoing cell division	

Signal Transduction Inhibitors	Chlorambucil	*Forms DNA cross-links and interferes with DNA replication	
	Cyclosporin	*Binds cyclophilin and prevents activation of calcineurin that is involved in the pathway of synthesis of IL-2 T-cell activation	NCT00001737 NCT00404482
	Tacrolimus	*Binds FK-506 binding protein 12 to create a complex that interferes with activity of calcineurin phosphatase and ultimately IL-2 and T-cell activity	
	Voclosporin	*Calcineurin inhibitor which inhibits IL-2 and T-cell activity	NCT01243983
	Sirolimus	*Macrolide antibiotic that binds FKBP-12 and inhibits the mTOR pathway *Inhibits the cell cycle and proliferation of T cells *Blunts IL-2 receptor and CD28-dependent signaling pathways *Blocks growth factor proliferation *Blocks activator of VEGF signaling	NCT00908466 NCT01280669

cases of uveitis and scleritis, more specifically in cases of ankylosing spondylitis and JIA.[93,94] Infliximab has been successful in the treatment of Behçet's disease and has been approved in Japan for this particular use.[95] One downside is it cannot be used intravitreally given adverse intraocular effects.

The remaining TNF-α targeting antibodies (adalimumab, certolizumab, golimumab) are all administered subcutaneously. Adalimumab (Humira, Abbott) is a fully human monoclonal antibody (mAb) and has been approved for several autoimmune diseases including rheumatoid arthritis, psoriatic arthritis, ankylosing spondylitis, Crohn's disease, JIA, and psoriasis. It is most commonly administered in 40 mg subcutaneous injections every 2 weeks. Studies have shown adalimumab to be affective in treatment of resistant uveitis,[96] JIA, Behçet's and ankylosing spondylitis-associated uveitis.[97–99] Adalimumab also has the potential for being used intravitreally as no adverse effects have been noted.[100]

The latest additions to this class of medications include certolizumab (Cimzia®, UCB S.A., Belgium) and golimumab (Simponi®, Centocor Biotech, Inc, PA). Golimumab is also a fully human mAb version of infliximab. It has been approved for rheumatoid arthritis, psoriatic arthritis, and ankylosing spondylitis. Only a few case reports have discussed the use of golimumab in the treatment of uveitis. One paper reports a possible efficacy and safety in treatment of refractory JIA-associated uveitis in three patients.[101] Certolizumab is unique in that it is comprised only of an antibody fragment complexed with PEG and is not an entire antibody, which leads to some limitations in its ability to fix complement or recruit antibody-dependent cell-mediated cytotoxicity. In 2008, the FDA-approved certolizumab for use in the US for treatment of Crohn's disease in patients non-responsive to other standard therapies. There has also been discussion for its use in treating rheumatoid arthritis. However, there have not been any reports regarding its use in treating ocular inflammatory disease.

Finally, it is important to note that inhibition of TNF-α function leaves patients susceptible to reactivation of tuberculosis, disseminated fungal disease, and other infections and may also have a greater risk of cancer and overall mortality.[70,102]

4.3.2.2. IL-2 receptor inhibitors

IL-2 is a cytokine essential for activation of T-lymphocytes. Daclizumab is a monoclonal antibody directed against the alpha subunit of the IL-2 receptor of activated T-lymphocytes. More specifically, it binds to the CD25 portion of the IL-2 receptor inhibiting the action of the IL-2-mediated cytokine response. Daclizumab has shown some significant promise in the treatment of childhood uveitis,[103] non-infectious intermediate and posterior uveitis[104] and refractory inflammatory disease.[105] It has also been particularly effective for birdshot retinochoroidopathy.[106,107] However, the manufacturer withdrew this medication from the market in January 2010 due to commercial reasons.

4.3.2.3. Rituximab

Rituximab or Rituxan® (Genentech, San Francisco, CA) is a chimeric anti-CD20 mAb. CD-20 is an antigenic marker found on the surfaces of B cells and is essential for activation and differentiation of B cells. In comparison to IL-2 inhibitors that primarily block T-lymphocytes, rituximab targets the humoral arm of the immune system. It is administered to patients who had an inadequate response to at least one TNF-α inhibitor by intravenous infusion. Rituximab has been a revolutionary therapy for the treatment of B-cell lymphoma. In addition, its applications have been expanding in the fields of rheumatology and ocular inflammatory disease. It was the first B-cell specific target for treatment of rheumatoid arthritis. In addition, in a multi-centered, randomized, blinded trial, rituximab was found to be non-inferior to cyclophosphamide, which is the standard of care in the treatment of ANCA-associated vasculitis.[108] Rituximab has also shown promising results in the field of ophthalmology in treating ocular cicatricial pemphigoid,[109] refractory Behçet's disease,[110] and orbital inflammatory syndrome.[111]

4.3.2.4. Abatacept

Abatacept or Orencia® (Bristol-Myers Squibb, New York, NY) is of the first approved agents in a class of medications that target T-cell co-stimulation signaling. T-cell co-stimulation involves two important steps. The first is the presentation of a processed antigen fragment by an MHC class II on an antigen-presenting cell to a T-cell receptor. The second step is the binding of the CD28 receptor on the T cell with CD86 or CD80 receptor on the antigen-presenting cell to complete co-stimulation. Abatacept is capable compromising important steps in co-stimulation by binding CD86/CD80 that is required for complete T-call activation.

Abatacept has been approved for the treatment of moderate to severe rheumatoid arthritis that have failed to improve on other therapies. Although abatacept is not currently approved for the treatment of uveitis, there is emerging data that suggests efficacy in the setting of recalcitrant JIA-associated uveitis that has failed traditional immune modulation or TNF inhibitors.[112]

4.3.2.5. IFN

Interferons are a group of cytokines synthesized by a variety of cell types that have immunomodulatory, antiviral, and anti-proliferative properties. The type 1 IFNs, which include IFN-α and $-\beta$ are most clinically relevant to ophthalmology. IFNs exert their immunomodulatory effects by increasing the expression of MHC class I on surface molecules and by the activation of macrophages and NK cells.

IFNs have been used in patients with a number of different ocular inflammatory disorders. It has been used in patients with ocular manifestations of Behçet's disease since 1994. In a non-controlled, open-label, prospective study of 50 patients with refractory Behçet's disease with ocular involvement treated with IFN-2α demonstrated a response rate of 92%, with significant improvements in visual acuity and ocular inflammation.[113] After an average of follow-up of 2.5 years, more than one third of the patients in this trial had completed therapy and were free of ocular inflammation. In addition, IFNs have also been positive results in patients with multiple sclerosis-associated uveitis treated with IFN-β_{1a}, symphathetic ophthalmia and idiopathic posterior uveitis (Table 6).[114–116]

Table 6. Immunomodulatory therapy — biologic response modifiers and their associated ophthalmic clinical trials.

Class	Drugs	Mechanism of Action	Clinical Trials Identifier	Notes
TNF-a inhibitors	Etanercept/ Enbrel®	Soluble, bivalent receptor to TNF-alpha	NCT00931957 NCT00001862	*FDA approved for treatment of rheumatoid, juvenile rheumatoid, and psoriatic arthritis.
	Infliximab/ Remicade®	Mouse human chimeric Ab to TNF-alpha	NCT00589628 NCT00273390	*FDA approved for treatment of ankylosing spondylitis, psoriatic and rheumatoid arthritis, Crohn's disease and ulcerative colitis, and psoriasis
	Adalimumab/ Humira®	Fully human monoclonal Ab to TNF-alpha	NCT01148225 NCT01385826 NCT01124838	*FDA approved for treatment of rheumatoid, juvenile rheumatoid and psoriatic arthritis, ankylosing spondylitis, and Crohn's disease
	Certolizumab/ Cimzia®	PEGylated Fab' fragment of a fully human Ab to TNF-alpha		*Most active clinical trials directed toward use in Crohns disease, UC, RA
	Golimumab/ Simponi®	Human monoclonal Ab to TNF-alpha		*Most active clinical trials directed toward use in RA, AS, UC
IL-2 receptor inhibitors	Daclizumab/ Zenapax®	Monoclonal Ab to alpha subunit of IL-2 receptor of activated T cells	NCT00043667 NCT00070759 NCT00130637	*Most often used for prevention of rejection of organ transplants, especially kidney transplants.

(Continued)

Table 6. *(Continud)*

Class	Drugs	Mechanism of Action	Clinical Trials Identifier	Notes
Chimeric anti-CD20 antibody	Rituximab/ Rituxan®	Chimeric Ab to CD20 on B cells	NCT00664599	*Most often used to treat leukemias and lymphomas, autoimmune disease ad anti-rejection treatment in organ transplant.
Inhibitors of CD86/ CD80 and T-cell activation	Abatacept/ Orencia®	Binds CD86/CD80 on antigen-presenting cells inhibiting T cell activation	NCT01279954 NCT01693640	*Approved for use in patients with RA that have failed other treatments.
Interferon	Interferon-alpha Interferon-beta	Increase expression of MHC Class I	NCT00344253	*Used in treatment of autoimmune diseases, skin cancers and papillomas, hematological malignancy, and hepatitis B and C.

5. Ongoing Clinical Trials and Potential Future Therapeutic Approaches

There are a number of medications currently being studied or discussed for the treatment of ocular inflammation. Many of these medications are already available for the treatment of other inflammatory diseases. Below we will discuss some of the potential future therapeutic approaches for the treatment of ocular inflammation and will list some of the clinical trials that have evaluated these medications (Table 7).

Tocilizumab or Actemra® (Genentech, San Francisco, CA) is a humanized antibody to IL-6, which is an important cytokine in the stimulation of B-cell and T-cell activation and differentiation. Tocilizumab is approved for use in treating moderate to severe rheumatoid arthritis or in patients who had inadequate responses to TNF-α inhibitors. It is dosed at 4–8 mg/kg intravenous infusion every 4 weeks. One of the greatest benefits is that due to its target of IL-6, the concern of reactivation of tuberculosis is less of an issue compared to other biologics. There has only been one case report using Tocilizumab to treat ocular inflammatory disease. The report states treatment success in a patient with refractory uveitis in the setting of Castleman's disease.[117]

Anakinra or Kinerset® (Amgen, Thousand Oaks, CA) is a human recombinant IL-1 receptor antagonist. IL-1 is a cytokine that stimulates inflammation and the recruitment of inflammatory cells to a particular tissue site. Given that IL-1 has been implicated in inflammatory diseases such as rheumatoid arthritis, Anakinra has been approved for use in patients with rheumatoid arthritis. Application of this medication includes a 100 mg subcutaneous injection daily. There is limited data in the use of Anakinra in the use of ocular inflammatory disease. However, there have been case reports of its use in refractory Behçet's disease, chronic infantile neurological cutaneous articular syndrome (CINCA)-associated uveitis[118] and JIA. A multicenter trial has demonstrated its efficacy in its use as a first-line agent in JIA treatment.[119]

Ustekinumab or Stelera® (Centocor Biotech, Inc, PA) is a fully human immunoglobulin with targets both IL-12 and IL-23. These two cytokines are implicated in psoriasis. Ustekinumab is administered subcutaneously and is dosed at 45 mg (if weight < 100 kg) and 90 mg (if weight > 100 kg)

Table 7. Other novel ocular immunomodulatory therapies and ophthalmic clinical trials.

Drug	Company	Mechanism of Action	Indications	Clinical Phase	Clinical Trials Identifier
Secukinumab (AIN457)	Novartis	Human monoclonal IL-17A Ab	Noninfectious uveitis, psoriasis, rheumatoid arthritis, ankylosing spondylitis	II, III	NCT00685399 NCT00995709 NCt01090310 (SHIELD, INSURE ENDURE)
Tocilizumab (Actemra®)	Hoffman-La Roche and Chugai	Humanized Ab to IL-6	Rheumatoid arthritis, non-infectious uveitis, refractory uveitis	I,II	NCT0171710 NCT00348153
Anakinra (Kineret®)	Amgen	Human recombinant IL-1 receptor antagonist	Rheumatoid arthritis, Behcet's disease, JIA, CINCA-associated uveitis	I, II	NCT01441076
Ustekinumab (Stelera®)	Centocor and Janssen-Cilag	Human Ab to IL-12 and IL-23	Psoriasis, Crohn's disease, rheumatoid arthritis,	I, II	NCT01647152
Alemtuzumab (Campath®, Lemtrada®)	Genzyme/ Sanofi	Anti-CD52 Ab (T-cell selective)	CLL, Hodgkin's disease, preventing graft rejection		
Basiliximab (Simulect®)	Novartis	Monoclonal anti-CD25/ IL-2 Ab	Preventing graft rejection, keratoplasty, noninfectious uveitis	II	NCT00409656 NCT00646425

Apremilast	Celgene	Inhibitor of phosphodiesterase IV/ TNF-a	Psoriatic arthritis, Behcet's disease, rheumatoid arthritis, ankylosing spondylitis, rosacea		NCT00866359 NCT01045551
ESBA-105	Alcon	Anti-TNF-a Ab	Acute anterior uveitis, dry eye syndrome	II	NCT00823173 NCT00820014 NCT01338610
MM-093	Merrimack	Recombinant human alpha-fetoprotein	Rheumatoid arthritis, psoriasis, uveitis	II	NCT00444743
EGP-437	EyeGate Pharma	Dexamethasone phosphate	Dry eye, anterior uveitis, cataract surgery, scleritis	II, III	NCT01129856 NCT00694135 NCT01602068 NCT00765804 NCT01059955
Bevacizumab (Avastin™)	Genentech	Anti-VEGF monoclonal Ab	Ocular inflammation, diabetic macular edema, ARMD, CME	II, III	NCT0040712 NCT01823081
Ranibizumab (Lucentis™)	Genentech	Anti-VEGF monoclonal Ab	Ocular inflammation, diabetic macular edema, ARMD, CME, RVO	I, II	NCT00498355 NCT01564108
Everolimus (Zortress®, Certican®, Afinitor®)	Novartis	mTOR inhibitor	Prevention of graft rejection, tumor treatment like RCC	II	NCT00803816

(Continud)

Table 7. (*Continud*)

Drug	Company	Mechanism of Action	Indications	Clinical Phase	Clinical Trials Identifier
Canakinumab (Ilaris®)	Novartis	Monoclonal IL-1B Ab	JIA, Gout		
B27PD (Optiquel®)		B27PD protein fragment	Non-infectious uveitis	I, II	NCT01195948
Cyclosporin Implant	NEI	Inhibits production of IL-2	Uveitis	I	NCT00001737
Interferon Gamma -1b	NEI	Interferon Gamma -1b	CME secondary to uveitis	I, II	NCT01376362
Efalizumab	NEI		Uveitis	I	NCT00280826
Gevokizumab	XOMA LLC		Non-infectious uveitis	I	NCT01684345
Intravitreal Methotrexate	NEI	Inhibits DHFR and DNA synthesis	Non-infectious Intermediate and Posterior uveitis, macular edema	I, II	NCT01314417

every 12 weeks after a 2-doses loading spaced out by 4 weeks. Given that there are no significant data related to ocular therapy, studies need to be initiated in order to determine if this medication is of benefit in the treatment of ocular inflammatory disorders.

AIN457 is a monoclonal antibody, which inhibits IL-17 and is secreted by Th-17 cells. IL-17 has evolved as a key mediator in autoimmune disease. AIN457 is under development by Novartis for the treatment of psoriasis, uveitis, and other inflammatory diseases and is currently in Phase III trials.

Alemtuzumab or Campath® or Lamtrada® (Genzyme or Sanofi, S.A., Paris, France) is a humanized anti-CD52 antibody and offers an alternative T-cell selective agent that could be of benefit in treatment ocular inflammatory disease. It is given intravenously over 5 consecutive days. The downfalls of this medication include pan-lymphocyte depletion with profound lymphopenia.

Basiliximab or Simulect® (Novartis, Basel, Switzerland) is a chimeric monoclonal antibody against CD25 for renal allograft rejection. It may be an alternative agent to daclizumab, now that this medication is off the market.

Apremilast is a selective cytokine inhibitory drug under development by Celgene (Summit, NJ) that inhibits phosphodiesterase IV and thereby inhibits TNF-α. The greatest benefit of this drug is its ability to provide an oral medication, whereas all other TNF-α inhibitors are administered subcutaneously or intravenously. It is currently being studied in psoriasis, Behçet's disease, and rheumatoid arthritis, but not uveitis.

ESBA-105 is an anti-TNF-α single chain antibody under development by Alcon. It is administered topically, which would be of great benefit in avoiding systemic side effects. ESBA-105 is being evaluated for use in ocular conditions including uveitis, diabetic retinopathy, and AMD. So far, it has shown good ocular anterior and posterior penetration.[120]

MM-093 is a recombinant human alpha-fetoprotein under development by Merrimack (Cambridge, MA) for multiple autoimmune disorders. Clinical trials using MM-093 have evaluated its use in patients with sarcoidosis and birdshot uveitis.

EGP-437 is a formulation of dexamethasone phosphate under development by EyeGate Pharma (Waltham, MA) for the treatment of uveitis and dry eye. Study results available thus far have shown a statistically significant improvement in dry eye syndrome.[121]

Bevacizumab (Avastin™, Genentech, San Francisco, CA) and ranibizumab (Lucentis™, Genentech Inc, San Francisco, CA) are both monoclonal antibodies that inhibit vascular endothelial growth factor (VEGF). Ranibizumab was specifically designed for ocular use and received FDA approval for the treatment of choroidal neovascularization in AMD, while bevacizumab is FDA approved for colorectal cancer, but is currently used off-label very regularly for use in ocular disease. Previous studies have showed increased levels of VEGF in the aqueous humor of the eye in patients with uveitis and CME, compared to eyes with uveitis without CME.[122] In a prospective, case series of six patients with quiet uveitis with CME refractory to standard therapy, ranibizumab was given monthly for 3 months followed by re-injection as needed. Both vision and central retinal thickness improved at 3 and 6 months with adverse effects noted (Table 7).[123]

6. Conclusion

The ultimate goal of uveitis therapy is to induce drug-free remission of the disease. Unfortunately, in severe disease only a few drugs can reach this level of success. Currently, success in uveitis therapy is more often defined by treatments that are able to maintain a relative level of quiescence, drug-free periods, and the ability to taper the dosage of steroids. More often than not, more than one agent is needed to achieve durable remission.

Our advancements in the understanding of immunological diseases have provided many opportunities for the development of novel therapies and drug delivery systems. However, there are still many questions to be answered and many opportunities for drug development. Further interventional and longitudinal studies must be done to evaluate each of these medications impact on treatment of inflammatory disease, and more specifically in this case, ocular inflammatory disease.

7. References

1. Suttorp-Schulten, M.S., Rothova, A. The possible impact of uveitis in blindness: a literature survey. *Br J Ophthalmol* [Review] **80**(9), 844–848 (1996).

2. Rothova, A., Suttorp-van Schulten, M.S., Frits Treffers, W., Kijlstra, A. Causes and frequency of blindness in patients with intraocular inflammatory disease. *Br J Ophthalmol* **80**(4), 332–336 (1996).
3. Jabs, D.A., Nussenblatt, R.B., Rosenbaum, J.T. Standardization of uveitis nomenclature for reporting clinical data. Results of the First International Workshop. *Am J Ophthalmol* [Research Support, Non-U.S. Gov't Review] **140**(3), 509–516 (2005).
4. Flach, A.J. Topical nonsteroidal antiinflammatory drugs in ophthalmology. Int *Ophthalmol Clin.* [Research Support, Non-U.S. Gov't Research Support, U.S. Gov't, Non-P.H.S. Research Support, U.S. Gov't, P.H.S. Review] **42**(1), 1–11 (2002).
5. Flach, A.J. Cyclo-oxygenase inhibitors in ophthalmology. *Surv Ophthalmol* [Review] **36**(4), 259–284 (1992).
6. Kim, S.J., Flach, A.J., Jampol, L.M. Nonsteroidal anti-inflammatory drugs in ophthalmology. *Surv Ophthalmol* [Research Support, Non-U.S. Gov't Review] **55**(2), 108–133 (2010).
7. Snir, M., Axer-Siegel, R., Friling, R., Weinberger, D. Efficacy of diclofenac versus dexamethasone for treatment after strabismus surgery. *Ophthalmology* [Clinical Trial Comparative Study Randomized Controlled Trial] **107**(10), 1884–1888 (2000).
8. Wright, M., Butt, Z., McIlwaine, G., Fleck, B. Comparison of the efficacy of diclofenac and betamethasone following strabismus surgery. *Br J Ophthalmol* [Clinical Trial Comparative Study Randomized Controlled Trial] **81**(4), 299–301 (1997).
9. Mirshahi, A., Djalilian, A., Rafiee, F., Namavari, A. Topical administration of diclofenac (1%) in the prevention of miosis during vitrectomy. *Retina* [Randomized Controlled Trial] **28**(9), 1215–1220 (2008).
10. Kim, S.J., Lo, W.R., Hubbard, G.B., 3rd, Srivastava, S.K., Denny, J.P., Martin, D.F., *et al.* Topical ketorolac in vitreoretinal surgery: a prospective, randomized, placebo-controlled, double-masked trial. *Arch Ophthalmol* [Randomized Controlled Trial Research Support, Non-U.S. Gov't] **126**(9), 1203–1208 (2008).
11. Herbort, C.P., Mermoud, A., Schnyder, C., Pittet, N. Anti-inflammatory effect of diclofenac drops after argon laser trabeculoplasty. *Arch Ophthalmol* [Clinical Trial Randomized Controlled Trial] **111**(4), 481–483 (1993).
12. Hotchkiss, M.L., Robin, A.L., Pollack, I.P., Quigley, H.A. Nonsteroidal anti-inflammatory agents after argon laser trabeculoplasty. A trial with

flurbiprofen and indomethacin. *Ophthalmology* [Clinical Trial Comparative Study Randomized Controlled Trial]. **91**(8), 969–976 (1984).

13. Hurvitz, L.M., Spaeth, G.L., Zakhour, I., Mahmood, E., Murray, G. A comparison of the effect of flurbiprofen, dexamethasone, and placebo on cyclocryotherapy-induced inflammation. *Ophthalmic Surg* [Clinical Trial Comparative Study Randomized Controlled Trial Research Support, Non-U.S. Gov't] **15**(5), 394–399 (1984).

14. Dunne, J.A., Jacobs, N., Morrison, A., Gilbert, D.J. Efficacy in anterior uveitis of two known steroids and topical tolmetin. *Br J Ophthalmol* [Clinical Trial Comparative Study Randomized Controlled Trial] **69**(2), 120–125 (1985).

15. Young, B.J., Cunningham, W.F., Akingbehin, T. Double-masked controlled clinical trial of 5% tolmetin versus 0.5% prednisolone versus 0.9% saline in acute endogenous nongranulomatous anterior uveitis. *Br J Ophthalmol* [Clinical Trial Comparative Study Randomized Controlled Trial] **66**(6), 389–391 (1982).

16. Rabiah, P.K., Fiscella, R.G., Tessler, H.H. Intraocular penetration of periocular ketorolac and efficacy in experimental uveitis. *Invest Ophthalmol Vis Sci* [Research Support, Non-U.S. Gov't] **37**(4), 613–618 (1996).

17. Noble, A.G., Tripathi, R.C., Levine, R.A. Indomethacin for the treatment of idiopathic orbital myositis. *Am J Ophthalmol* [Case Reports] **108**(3), 336–338 (1989).

18. Jabs, D.A., Mudun, A., Dunn, J.P., Marsh, M.J. Episcleritis and scleritis: clinical features and treatment results. *Am J Ophthalmol* **130**(4), 469–476 (2000).

19. Tuft, S.J., Watson, P.G. Progression of scleral disease. *Ophthalmology* **98**(4), 467–471 (1991).

20. Watson, P.G., Hayreh, S.S. Scleritis and episcleritis. *Br J Ophthalmol* **60**(3), 163–191 (1976).

21. Yeh, S., Faia, L.J., Nussenblatt, R.B. Advances in the diagnosis and immunotherapy for ocular inflammatory disease. *Semin Immunopathol* [Review] **30**(2), 145–164 (2008).

22. Diestelhorst, M., Aspacher, F., Konen, W., Krieglstein, G.K., Hilgers, R.D. Effect of 0.1% dexamethasone and 1.0% prednisolone acetate eyedrops on the blood-aqueous humor barrier. *Ophthalmologe* [Clinical Trial Comparative Study Randomized Controlled Trial] **89**(4), 342–345 (1992).

23. Gaudio, P.A. A review of evidence guiding the use of corticosteroids in the treatment of intraocular inflammation. *Ocul Immunol Inflamm* [Research Support, Non-U.S. Gov't Review] **12**(3), 169–192 (2004).

24. Foster, C.S., Alter, G., DeBarge, L.R., Raizman, M.B., Crabb, J.L., Santos C.I., *et al*. Efficacy and safety of rimexolone 1% ophthalmic suspension vs 1% prednisolone acetate in the treatment of uveitis. *Am J Ophthalmol* [Clinical Trial Comparative Study Multicenter Study Randomized Controlled Trial Research Support, Non-U.S. Gov't] **122**(2), 171–182 (1996).

25. Controlled evaluation of loteprednol etabonate and prednisolone acetate in the treatment of acute anterior uveitis. Loteprednol Etabonate US Uveitis Study Group. *Am J Ophthalmol* [Clinical Trial Comparative Study Multicenter Study Randomized Controlled Trial Research Support, Non-U.S. Gov't] **127**(5), 537–544 (1999).

26. Bikowski, J., Pillai, R., Shroot, B. The position not the presence of the halogen in corticosteroids influences potency and side effects. *J Drugs Dermatol* [Review] **5**(2), 125–130 (2006).

27. Hammer, S., Spika, I., Sippl, W., Jessen, G., Kleuser, B., Holtje, H.D., *et al*. Glucocorticoid receptor interactions with glucocorticoids: evaluation by molecular modeling and functional analysis of glucocorticoid receptor mutants. *Steroids* [Comparative Study Research Support, Non-U.S. Gov't] **68**(4), 329–339 (2003).

28. Korenfeld, M.S., Silverstein, S.M., Cooke, D.L., Vogel, R., Crockett, R.S. Difluprednate ophthalmic emulsion 0.05% for postoperative inflammation and pain. *J Cataract Refract Surg* [Clinical Trial, Phase III Multicenter Study Randomized Controlled Trial Research Support, Non-U.S. Gov't] **35**(1), 26–34 (2009).

29. Foster, C.S., Davanzo, R., Flynn, T.E., McLeod, K., Vogel, R., Crockett, R.S. Durezol (Difluprednate Ophthalmic Emulsion 0.05%) compared with Pred Forte 1% ophthalmic suspension in the treatment of endogenous anterior uveitis. *J Ocul Pharmacol Ther* [Clinical Trial, Phase III Comparative Study Randomized Controlled Trial Research Support, Non-U.S. Gov't] **26**(5), 475–483 (2010).

30. Lyon, F., Gale, R.P., Lightman, S. Recent developments in the treatment of uveitis: an update. *Expert Opin Investig Drugs* [Review] **18**(5), 609–616 (2009).

31. Wakefield, D., McCluskey, P. Systemic immunosuppression in the treatment of posterior uveitis. *Int Ophthalmol Clin* [Review] **35**(3), 107–122 (1995).

32. Lightman, S. Uveitis: Management. *Lancet* [Review] 14;**338**(8781), 1501–1504 (1991).

33. Weijtens, O., Schoemaker, R.C., Cohen, A.F., Romijn, F.P., Lentjes, E.G., van Rooij, J., *et al.* Dexamethasone concentration in vitreous and serum after oral administration. *Am J Ophthalmol* [Comparative Study Research Support, Non-U.S. Gov't] **125**(5), 673–679 (1998).

34. Behar-Cohen, F.F., Gauthier, S., El Aouni, A., Chapon, P., Parel, J.M., Renard, G., *et al.* Methylprednisolone concentrations in the vitreous and the serum after pulse therapy. *Retina* [Research Support, Non-U.S. Gov't] **21**(1), 48–53 (2001).

35. Sherif, Z., Pleyer, U. Corticosteroids in ophthalmology: past-present-future. *Ophthalmologica* [Review] **216**(5), 305–315 (2002).

36. Lightman, S., Kok, H. Developments in the treatment of uveitis. *Expert Opin Investig Drugs* [Review] **11**(1), 59–67 (2002).

37. Wakefield, D., McCluskey, P., Penny, R. Intravenous pulse methylprednisolone therapy in severe inflammatory eye disease. *Arch Ophthalmol* [Case Reports Clinical Trial] **104**(6), 847–851 (1986).

38. Visual function 5 years after optic neuritis: experience of the Optic Neuritis Treatment Trial. The Optic Neuritis Study Group. *Arch Ophthalmol* [Clinical Trial Multicenter Study Randomized Controlled Trial Research Support, U.S. Gov't, P.H.S.] **115**(12), 1545–1552 (1997).

39. Toker, E., Kazokoglu, H., Acar, N. High dose intravenous steroid therapy for severe posterior segment uveitis in Behcet's disease. *Br J Ophthalmol* [Case Reports] **86**(5), 521–523 (2002).

40. Markomichelakis, N.N., Halkiadakis, I., Papaeythymiou-Orchan, S., Giannakopoulos, N., Ekonomopoulos, N., Kouris T. Intravenous pulse methylprednisolone therapy for acute treatment of serpiginous choroiditis. *Ocul Immunol Inflamm* [Case Reports] **14**(1), 29–33 (2006).

41. Helm, C.J., Holland, G.N. The effects of posterior subtenon injection of triamcinolone acetonide in patients with intermediate uveitis. *Am J Ophthalmol* [Research Support, Non-U.S. Gov't] **120**(1), 55–64 (1995).

42. Ferrante, P., Ramsey, A., Bunce, C., Lightman, S. Clinical trial to compare efficacy and side-effects of injection of posterior sub-Tenon triamcinolone versus orbital floor methylprednisolone in the management of posterior uveitis. *Clin Experiment Ophthalmol* [Clinical Trial Comparative Study Controlled Clinical Trial] **32**(6), 563–568 (2004).

43. Riordan-Eva, P., Lightman, S. Orbital floor steroid injections in the treatment of uveitis. *Eye (Lond)* **8**(Pt 1), 66–69 (1994).

44. Roesel, M., Heinz, C., Koch, J.M., Heiligenhaus, A. Comparison of orbital floor triamcinolone acetonide and oral prednisolone for cataract surgery management in patients with non-infectious uveitis. *Graefes Arch Clin Exp*

Ophthalmol [Comparative Study Randomized Controlled Trial] **248**(5), 715–720 (2010).

45. Nan, K., Sun, S., Li, Y., Qu, J., Li, G., Luo, L., *et al.* Characterisation of systemic and ocular drug level of triamcinolone acetonide following a single sub-Tenon injection. *Br J Ophthalmol* **94**(5), 654–658 (2010).

46. Kozak, I., Kayikcioglu, O.R., Cheng, L., Falkenstein, I., Silva, G.A., Yu, D.X., *et al.* The effect of recombinant human hyaluronidase on dexamethasone penetration into the posterior segment of the eye after sub-Tenon's injection. *J Ocul Pharmacol Ther* [Evaluation Studies] **22**(5), 362–369 (2006).

47. Inoue, M., Takeda, K., Morita, K., Yamada, M., Tanigawara, Y., Oguchi, Y. Vitreous concentrations of triamcinolone acetonide in human eyes after intravitreal or subtenon injection. *Am J Ophthalmol* [Comparative Study] **138**(6), 1046–1048 (2004).

48. Kosobucki, B.R., Freeman, W.R., Cheng, L. Photographic estimation of the duration of high dose intravitreal triamcinolone in the vitrectomised eye. *Br J Ophthalmol* [Research Support, N.I.H., Extramural] **90**(6), 705–708 (2006).

49. Jonas, J.B., Degenring, R., Kreissig, I., Akkoyun, I. Safety of intravitreal high-dose reinjections of triamcinolone acetonide. *Am J Ophthalmol* **138**(6), 1054–1055 (2004).

50. Maca, S.M., Abela-Formanek, C., Kiss, C.G., Sacu, S.G., Benesch, T., Barisani-Asenbauer, T. Intravitreal triamcinolone for persistent cystoid macular oedema in eyes with quiescent uveitis. *Clin Experiment Ophthalmol* **37**(4), 389–396 (2009).

51. Tuncer, S., Yilmaz, S., Urgancioglu, M., Tugal-Tutkun, I. Results of intra-vitreal triamcinolone acetonide (IVTA) injection for the treatment of panu-veitis attacks in patients with Behcet disease. *J Ocul Pharmacol Ther* **23**(4), 395–401 (2007).

52. Kramer, M., Ehrlich, R., Snir, M., Friling, R., Mukamel, M., Weinberger, D., *et al.* Intravitreal injections of triamcinolone acetonide for severe vitritis in patients with incomplete Behcet's disease. *Am J Ophthalmol* [Case Reports] **138**(4), 666–667 (2004).

53. Ozdemir, H., Karacorlu, M., Karacorlu, S. Intravitreal triamcinolone ace-tonide in sympathetic ophthalmia. *Graefes Arch Clin Exp Ophthalmol* [Case Reports] **243**(7), 734–736 (2005).

54. Chan, R.V., Seiff, B.D., Lincoff, H.A., Coleman, D.J. Rapid recovery of sympathetic ophthalmia with treatment augmented by intravitreal steroids. *Retina* [Case Reports] **26**(2), 243–247 (2006).

55. Karacorlu, M., Arf Karacorlu, S., Ozdemir, H. Intravitreal triamcinolone acetonide in Vogt-Koyanagi-Harada syndrome. *Eur J Ophthalmol* [Case Reports] **16**(3), 481–483 (2006).

56. Driot, J.Y., Novack, G.D., Rittenhouse, K.D., Milazzo, C., Pearson, P.A. Ocular pharmacokinetics of fluocinolone acetonide after Retisert intravitreal implantation in rabbits over a 1-year period. *J Ocul Pharmacol Ther* **20**(3), 269–275 (2004).

57. Mruthyunjaya, P., Khalatbari, D., Yang, P., Stinnett, S., Tano, R., Ashton, P., *et al.* Efficacy of low-release-rate fluocinolone acetonide intravitreal implants to treat experimental uveitis. *Arch Ophthalmol* [Research Support, N.I.H., Extramural Research Support, Non-U.S. Gov't] **124**(7), 1012–1018 (2006).

58. Kempen, J.H., Altaweel, M.M., Holbrook, J.T., Jabs, D.A., Sugar, E.A. The multicenter uveitis steroid treatment trial: rationale, design, and baseline characteristics. *Am J Ophthalmol* [Comparative Study Multicenter Study Randomized Controlled Trial] **149**(4), 550–561 e10 (2010).

59. Kempen, J.H., Altaweel, M.M., Holbrook, J.T., Jabs, D.A., Louis, T.A., Sugar, E.A., *et al.* Randomized comparison of systemic anti-inflammatory therapy versus fluocinolone acetonide implant for intermediate, posterior, and panuveitis: the multicenter uveitis steroid treatment trial. Ophthalmology [Comparative Study Multicenter Study Randomized Controlled Trial Research Support, N.I.H., Extramural Research Support, Non-U.S. Gov't] **118**(10), 1916–1926 (2011).

60. Callanan, D.G., Jaffe, G.J., Martin, D.F., Pearson, P.A., Comstock, T.L. Treatment of posterior uveitis with a fluocinolone acetonide implant: three-year clinical trial results. *Arch Ophthalmol* [Multicenter Study Randomized Controlled Trial Research Support, Non-U.S. Gov't] **126**(9), 1191–1201 (2008).

61. Jaffe, G.J., McCallum, R.M., Branchaud, B., Skalak, C., Butuner, Z., Ashton P. Long-term follow-up results of a pilot trial of a fluocinolone acetonide implant to treat posterior uveitis. *Ophthalmology* [Clinical Trial Randomized Controlled Trial Research Support, N.I.H., Extramural Research Support, Non-U.S. Gov't Research Support, U.S. Gov't, P.H.S.] **112**(7), 1192–1198 (2005).

62. Chieh, J.J., Carlson, A.N., Jaffe, G.J. Combined fluocinolone acetonide intraocular delivery system insertion, phacoemulsification, and intraocular lens implantation for severe uveitis. *Am J Ophthalmol* [Clinical Trial] **146**(4), 589–594 (2008).

63. Goldstein, D.A., Godfrey, D.G., Hall, A., Callanan, D.G., Jaffe, G.J., Pearson P.A., *et al.* Intraocular pressure in patients with uveitis treated with fluocinolone acetonide implants. *Arch Ophthalmol* [Research Support, Non-U.S. Gov't] **125**(11), 1478–1485 (2007).

64. Haller, J.A., Bandello, F., Belfort, R., Jr., Blumenkranz, M.S., Gillies, M., Heier, J., *et al.* Randomized, sham-controlled trial of dexamethasone intra-vitreal implant in patients with macular edema due to retinal vein occlusion. *Ophthalmology* [Multicenter Study Randomized Controlled Trial] **117**(6), 1134–1146 e3 (2010).

65. Kuppermann, B.D., Blumenkranz, M.S., Haller, J.A., Williams, G.A., Weinberg, D.V., Chou, C., *et al.* Randomized controlled study of an intra-vitreous dexamethasone drug delivery system in patients with persistent macular edema. *Arch Ophthalmol* [Multicenter Study Randomized Controlled Trial Research Support, Non-U.S. Gov't] **125**(3), 309–317 (2007).

66. Williams, G.A., Haller, J.A., Kuppermann, B.D., Blumenkranz, M.S., Weinberg, D.V., Chou, C., *et al.* Dexamethasone posterior-segment drug delivery system in the treatment of macular edema resulting from uveitis or Irvine-Gass syndrome. *Am J Ophthalmol* [Multicenter Study Randomized Controlled Trial Research Support, Non-U.S. Gov't] **147**(6), 1048–1054, 54 e1-2 (2009).

67. Siddique, S.S., Shah, R., Suelves, A.M., Foster, C.S. Road to remission: A comprehensive review of therapy in uveitis. *Expert Opin Investig Drugs* [Review] **20**(11), 1497–1515 (2011).

68. Campochiaro, P.A., Hafiz, G., Shah, S.M., Bloom, S., Brown, D.M., Busquets, M., *et al.* Sustained ocular delivery of fluocinolone acetonide by an intravitreal insert. *Ophthalmology* [Clinical Trial, Phase II Comparative Study Multicenter Study Randomized Controlled Trial Research Support, Non-U.S. Gov't] **117**(7), 1393–1399 e3 (2010).

69. Gangaputra, S., Newcomb, C.W., Liesegang, T.L., Kacmaz, R.O., Jabs, D.A., Levy-Clarke, GA., *et al.* Methotrexate for ocular inflammatory diseases. *Ophthalmology* [Multicenter Study Research Support, N.I.H., Extramural Research Support, Non-U.S. Gov't] **116**(11), 2188–2198 e1 (2009).

70. Kempen, J.H., Daniel, E., Dunn, J.P., Foster, C.S., Gangaputra, S., Hanish, A., *et al.* Overall and cancer related mortality among patients with ocular inflammation treated with immunosuppressive drugs: retrospective cohort study. *BMJ* [Multicenter Study Research Support, N.I.H., Extramural

Research Support, N.I.H., Intramural Research Support, Non-U.S. Gov't]
339, b2480 (2009).

71. Lee, F.F., Foster, C.S. Pharmacotherapy of uveitis. *Expert Opin Pharmacother* [Review] **11**(7), 1135–1146 (2010).

72. Newell, F.W., Krill, A.E. Treatment of uveitis with azathioprine (Imuran). *Trans Ophthalmol Soc U K* **87**, 499–511 (1967).

73. Andrasch, R.H., Pirofsky, B., Burns, R.P. Immunosuppressive therapy for severe chronic uveitis. *Arch Ophthalmol* **96**(2), 247–251 (1978).

74. Baltatzis, S., Tufail, F., Yu, E.N., Vredeveld, C.M., Foster, C.S. Mycophenolate mofetil as an immunomodulatory agent in the treatment of chronic ocular inflammatory disorders. *Ophthalmology* **110**(5), 1061–1065 (2003).

75. Daniel, E., Thorne, J.E., Newcomb, C.W., Pujari, S.S., Kacmaz, R.O., Levy-Clarke, GA., *et al.* Mycophenolate mofetil for ocular inflammation. *Am J Ophthalmol* [Multicenter Study Research Support, N.I.H., Extramural Research Support, Non-U.S. Gov't Research Support, U.S. Gov't, Non-P.H.S.] **149**(3), 423–432 e1-2 (2010).

76. Roda, E. Uveitis treated with nitrogen mustard. *Am J Ophthalmol* **35**(1), 114 (1952).

77. Brubaker, R., Font, R.L., Shepherd, E.M. Granulomatous sclerouveitis. Regression of ocular lesions with cyclophosphamide and prednisone. *Arch Ophthalmol* **86**(5), 517–524 (1971).

78. Fauci, A.S., Doppman, J.L., Wolff, S.M. Cyclophosphamide-induced remissions in advanced polyarteritis nodosa. *Am J Med* [Case Reports] **64**(5), 890–894 (1978).

79. Fosdick, W.M., Parsons, J.L., Hill, D.F. Long-term cyclophosphamide therapy in rheumatoid arthritis. *Arthritis Rheum* **11**(2), 151–161 (1968).

80. Hoang-Xaun, T., Foster, C.S., Rice, B.A. Scleritis in relapsing polychondritis. Response to therapy. *Ophthalmology* [Research Support, Non-U.S. Gov't] **97**(7), 892–898 (1990).

81. Austin, H.A., 3rd, Klippel, J.H., Balow, J.E., le Riche, N.G., Steinberg, A.D., Plotz, P.H., *et al.* Therapy of lupus nephritis. Controlled trial of prednisone and cytotoxic drugs. *N Engl J Med* [Clinical Trial Comparative Study Randomized Controlled Trial Research Support, Non-U.S. Gov't] **314**(10), 614–619 (1986).

82. Pujari, S.S., Kempen, J.H., Newcomb, C.W., Gangaputra, S., Daniel, E., Suhler, E.B., *et al.* Cyclophosphamide for ocular inflammatory diseases. *Ophthalmology* [Multicenter Study Research Support, N.I.H., Extramural Research Support, Non-U.S. Gov't] **117**(2), 356–365 (2010).

83. Mudun, B.A., Ergen, A., Ipcioglu, S.U., Burumcek, E.Y., Durlu, Y., Arslan, M.O. Short-term chlorambucil for refractory uveitis in Behcet's disease. *Ocul Immunol Inflamm* [Clinical Trial] **9**(4), 219–229 (2001).

84. Mochizuki, M., Masuda, K., Sakane, T., Ito, K., Kogure, M., Sugino, N., *et al.* A clinical trial of FK506 in refractory uveitis. *Am J Ophthalmol* [Clinical Trial Controlled Clinical Trial Multicenter Study] **115**(6), 763–769 (1993).

85. Murphy, C.C., Greiner, K., Plskova, J., Duncan, L., Frost, N.A., Forrester, J.V., *et al.* Cyclosporine vs tacrolimus therapy for posterior and intermediate uveitis. *Arch Ophthalmol* [Clinical Trial Comparative Study Multicenter Study Randomized Controlled Trial Research Support, Non-U.S. Gov't] **123**(5), 634–641 (2005).

86. Hogan, A.C., McAvoy, C.E., Dick, A.D., Lee, R.W. Long-term efficacy and tolerance of tacrolimus for the treatment of uveitis. *Ophthalmology* [Research Support, Non-U.S. Gov't] **114**(5), 1000–1006 (2007).

87. Anglade, E., Aspeslet, L.J., Weiss, S.L. A new agent for the treatment of noninfectious uveitis: rationale and design of three LUMINATE (Lux Uveitis Multicenter Investigation of a New Approach to Treatment) trials of steroid-sparing voclosporin. *Clin Ophthalmol* **2**(4), 693–702 (2008).

88. Roesel, M., Tappeiner, C., Heiligenhaus, A., Heinz, C. Oral voclosporin: novel calcineurin inhibitor for treatment of noninfectious uveitis. *Clin Ophthalmol* **5**, 1309–1313 (2011).

89. Nussenblatt, R.B., Coleman, H., Jirawuthiworavong, G., Davuluri, G., Potapova, N., Dahr, S.S., *et al.* The treatment of multifocal choroiditis associated choroidal neovascularization with sirolimus (rapamycin). *Acta Ophthalmol Scand* [Case Reports Letter] **85**(2), 230–231 (2007).

90. Shanmuganathan, V.A., Casely, E.M., Raj, D., Powell, R.J., Joseph, A., Amoaku, W.M., *et al.* The efficacy of sirolimus in the treatment of patients with refractory uveitis. *Br J Ophthalmol* [Clinical Trial] **89**(6), 666–669 (2005).

91. Foster, C.S., Tufail, F., Waheed, N.K., Chu, D., Miserocchi, E., Baltatzis, S., *et al.* Efficacy of etanercept in preventing relapse of uveitis controlled by methotrexate. *Arch Ophthalmol* [Clinical Trial Comparative Study Evaluation Studies Randomized Controlled Trial] **121**(4), 437–440 (2003).

92. Wendling, D., Paccou, J., Berthelot, J.M., Flipo, R.M., Guillaume-Czitrom, S., Prati, C., *et al.* New onset of uveitis during anti-tumor

necrosis factor treatment for rheumatic diseases. *Semin Arthritis Rheum* **41**(3), 503–510 (2011).

93. Breban, M., Vignon, E., Claudepierre, P., Devauchelle, V., Wendling, D., Lespessailles, E., *et al.* Efficacy of infliximab in refractory ankylosing spondylitis: results of a six-month open-label study. *Rheumatology (Oxford)* [Clinical Trial Multicenter Study] **41**(11), 1280–1285 (2002).

94. Mangge, H., Heinzl, B., Grubbauer, H.M., El-Shabrawi, Y., Schauenstein, K. Therapeutic experience with infliximab in a patient with polyarticular juvenile idiopathic arthritis and uveitis. *Rheumatol Int* [Case Reports] **23**(5), 258–261 (2003).

95. Arida, A., Fragiadaki, K., Giavri, E., Sfikakis, P.P. Anti-TNF agents for Behcet's disease: analysis of published data on 369 patients. *Semin Arthritis Rheum* [Research Support, Non-U.S. Gov't Review] **41**(1), 61–70 (2011).

96. Diaz-Llopis, M., Garcia-Delpech, S., Salom, D., Udaondo, P., Hernandez-Garfella, M., Bosch-Morell, F., *et al.* Adalimumab therapy for refractory uveitis: a pilot study. *J Ocul Pharmacol Ther* [Clinical Trial Research Support, Non-U.S. Gov't] **24**(3), 351–361 (2008).

97. Mushtaq, B., Saeed, T., Situnayake, R.D., Murray, P.I. Adalimumab for sight-threatening uveitis in Behcet's disease. *Eye (Lond)* [Case Reports] **21**(6), 824–825 (2007).

98. Takase, K., Ohno, S., Ideguchi, H., Uchio, E., Takeno, M., Ishigatsubo, Y. Successful switching to adalimumab in an infliximab-allergic patient with severe Behcet disease-related uveitis. *Rheumatol Int* [Case Reports] **31**(2), 243–245 (2011).

99. Biester, S., Deuter, C., Michels, H., Haefner, R., Kuemmerle-Deschner, J., Doycheva, D., *et al.* Adalimumab in the therapy of uveitis in childhood. *Br J Ophthalmol* [Multicenter Study] **91**(3), 319–324 (2007).

100. Androudi, S., Tsironi, E., Kalogeropoulos, C., Theodoridou, A., Brazitikos, P. Intravitreal adalimumab for refractory uveitis-related macular edema. *Ophthalmology* **117**(8), 1612–1616 (2010).

101. William, M., Faez, S., Papaliodis, G.N., Lobo, A.M. Golimumab for the treatment of refractory juvenile idiopathic arthritis-associated uveitis. *J Ophthalmic Inflamm Infect* **2**(4), 231–233 (2012).

102. Braun, J., Brandt, J., Listing, J., Zink, A., Alten, R., Burmester, G., *et al.* Long-term efficacy and safety of infliximab in the treatment of ankylosing spondylitis: an open, observational, extension study of a three-month, randomized, placebo-controlled trial. *Arthritis Rheum* [Clinical Trial

Randomized Controlled Trial Research Support, Non-U.S. Gov't] **48**(8), 2224–2233 (2003).

103. Gallagher, M., Quinones, K., Cervantes-Castaneda, R.A., Yilmaz, T., Foster C.S. Biological response modifier therapy for refractory childhood uveitis. *Br J Ophthalmol* [Evaluation Studies] **91**(10), 1341–1344 (2007).

104. Nussenblatt, R.B., Peterson, J.S., Foster, C.S., Rao, N.A., See. R.F., Letko E., *et al.* Initial evaluation of subcutaneous daclizumab treatments for noninfectious uveitis: a multicenter noncomparative interventional case series. *Ophthalmology* [Clinical Trial Multicenter Study Research Support, Non-U.S. Gov't Research Support, U.S. Gov't, P.H.S.] **112**(5), 764–770 (2005).

105. Bhat, P., Castaneda-Cervantes, R.A., Doctor, P.P., Foster, C.S. Intravenous daclizumab for recalcitrant ocular inflammatory disease. *Graefes Arch Clin Exp Ophthalmol* **247**(5), 687–692 (2009).

106. Kiss, S., Ahmed, M., Letko, E., Foster, C.S. Long-term follow-up of patients with birdshot retinochoroidopathy treated with corticosteroid-sparing systemic immunomodulatory therapy. *Ophthalmology* **112**(6), 1066–1071 (2005).

107. Sobrin, L., Huang, J.J., Christen, W., Kafkala, C., Choopong, P., Foster, C.S. Daclizumab for treatment of birdshot chorioretinopathy. *Arch Ophthalmol* **126**(2), 186–191 (2008).

108. Stone, J.H., Merkel, P.A., Spiera, R., Seo, P., Langford, C.A., Hoffman, G.S., *et al.* Rituximab versus cyclophosphamide for ANCA-associated vasculitis. *N Engl J Med* [Multicenter Study Randomized Controlled Trial Research Support, N.I.H., Extramural Research Support, Non-U.S. Gov't] **363**(3), 221–232 (2010).

109. Foster, C.S., Chang, P.Y., Ahmed, A.R. Combination of rituximab and intravenous immunoglobulin for recalcitrant ocular cicatricial pemphigoid: a preliminary report. *Ophthalmology* [Comparative Study] **117**(5), 861–869 (2010).

110. Davatchi, F., Shams, H., Rezaipoor, M., Sadeghi-Abdollahi, B., Shahram, F., Nadji, A., *et al.* Rituximab in intractable ocular lesions of Behcet's disease; randomized single-blind control study (pilot study). *Int J Rheum Dis* [Randomized Controlled Trial] **13**(3), 246–252 (2010).

111. Kurz, P.A., Suhler, E.B., Choi, D., Rosenbaum, J.T. Rituximab for treatment of ocular inflammatory disease: a series of four cases. *Br J Ophthalmol* [Case Reports Research Support, Non-U.S. Gov't] **93**(4), 546–548 (2009).

112. Kenawy, N., Cleary, G., Mewar, D., Beare, N., Chandna, A., Pearce, I. Abatacept: a potential therapy in refractory cases of juvenile idiopathic arthritis-associated uveitis. *Graefes Arch Clin Exp Ophthalmol* [Case Reports] **249**(2), 297–300 (2011).

113. Kotter, I., Vonthein, R., Zierhut, M., Eckstein, A.K., Ness, T., Gunaydin, I., *et al.* Differential efficacy of human recombinant interferon-alpha2a on ocular and extraocular manifestations of Behcet disease: results of an open 4-center trial. *Semin Arthritis Rheum* [Clinical Trial Multicenter Study] **33**(5), 311–319 (2004).

114. Mackensen, F., Max, R., Becker, M.D. Interferons and their potential in the treatment of ocular inflammation. *Clin Ophthalmol* 3, 559–566 (2009).

115. Bodaghi, B., Gendron, G., Wechsler, B., Terrada, C., Cassoux, N., Huong du, L.T., *et al.* Efficacy of interferon alpha in the treatment of refractory and sight threatening uveitis: a retrospective monocentric study of 45 patients. *Br J Ophthalmol* **91**(3), 335–339 (2007).

116. Plskova, J., Greiner, K., Forrester, J.V. Interferon-alpha as an effective treatment for noninfectious posterior uveitis and panuveitis. *Am J Ophthalmol* [Research Support, Non-U.S. Gov't] **144**(1), 55–61 (2007).

117. Oshitari, T., Kajita, F., Tobe, A., Itami, M., Yotsukura, J., Baba, T., *et al.* Refractory uveitis in patient with castleman disease successfully treated with tocilizumab. *Case Rep Ophthalmol Med* **2012**, 968180 (2012).

118. Imrie, F.R., Dick, A.D. Biologics in the treatment of uveitis. *Curr Opin Ophthalmol* [Review] **18**(6), 481–486 (2007).

119. Nigrovic, P.A., Mannion, M., Prince, F.H., Zeft, A., Rabinovich, C.E., van Rossum, M.A., *et al.* Anakinra as first-line disease-modifying therapy in systemic juvenile idiopathic arthritis: report of forty-six patients from an international multicenter series. *Arthritis Rheum* [Clinical Trial Multicenter Study Research Support, Non-U.S. Gov't] **63**(2), 545–555 (2011).

120. Ottiger, M., Thiel, M.A., Feige, U., Lichtlen, P., Urech, D.M. Efficient intraocular penetration of topical anti-TNF-alpha single-chain antibody (ESBA105) to anterior and posterior segment without penetration enhancer. *Invest Ophthalmol Vis Sci* **50**(2), 779–786 (2009).

121. Patane, M.A., Cohen, A., From, S., Torkildsen, G., Welch, D., Ousler, G.W., 3rd. Ocular iontophoresis of EGP-437 (dexamethasone phosphate) in dry eye patients: results of a randomized clinical trial. *Clin Ophthalmol* 5, 633–643 (2011).

122. Fine, H.F., Baffi, J., Reed, G.F., Csaky, K.G., Nussenblatt, R.B. Aqueous humor and plasma vascular endothelial growth factor in uveitis-associated cystoid macular edema. *Am J Ophthalmol* [Comparative Study] **132**(5), 794–796 (2001).

123. Acharya, N.R., Hong, K.C., Lee, S.M. Ranibizumab for refractory uveitis-related macular edema. *Am J Ophthalmol* [Research Support, N.I.H., Extramural] **148**(2), 303–309 e2 (2009).

Chapter 6: Nanoparticles for Ocular Drug Delivery

Qiangzhe Zhang, Jieming Li, Weiwei Gao and Liangfang Zhang

Department of NanoEngineering and Moores Cancer Center,
University of California, San Diego, La Jolla, CA 92093, USA

1. Introduction

The use of classic drug formulations to treat ocular diseases, including many vision threatening ones, has been challenged by the unique anatomical and physiological characteristics of the eye that restrict drug bioavailability.[1] Topical drugs in the form of eye drops, suspensions, and ointments are the preferred methods of administration to the anterior segment of the eyes, and these offer the advantages of easy practice and low cost. However, various clearance mechanisms present on the corneal surface, including lacrimation, tear dilution, and rapid tear turn-over, significantly limit the retention of drug molecules on the eye surface.[2] Meanwhile, the corneal epithelium imposes further protection through the presence of abundant tight junctions and desmosomes that effectively exclude foreign molecules and particles.[3,4] These barriers further limit the amount of drug molecules that is ultimately absorbed into the intraocular tissues.

At the same time, the administration of drugs to the posterior segment of the eyes is also challenging. Due to the lack of cellular components in the vitreous body, the convection of molecules to the posterior segment is significantly reduced. As the majority of blinding diseases are associated with this part of the eyes, efficient drug delivery strategies are urgently needed.[5] Systemic administration has been adopted to deliver drug molecules to the posterior segment of the eyes; however, the iris blood vessels and the non-pigmented layer of the ciliary epithelium constitute a blood-aqueous barrier, which limits the passage of molecules from the blood to the inner part of the eyes. Moreover, the retinal pigment epithelium (RPE), along with the endothelium of the retinal vessels, creates the inner and the outer blood-retina barriers that restrict the transport of molecules from the blood to the retina and vitreous cavity.[6] As a result, systemic administration often requires large and frequent doses, which are inevitably associated with poor patient compliance and increased risk of systemic side effects.

Recently, intravitreal injections and vitreal implants, despite their highly invasive nature, have been applied in order to achieve therapeutic concentrations of drug at the posterior segment. For example, intravitreal injection of drugs such as bevacizumab and ranibizumab are currently under investigation to treat vascular diseases associated with the posterior segment of the eyes, including choroidal neovascularization and retinopathy of prematurity.[7-9] It is clear that frequent administration through the intravitreal route is associated with short-term adverse effects such as retinal detachment, endophthalmitis, intravitreal hemorrhage, and increased risk of cataract development.[2] To address these challenges, periocular drug delivery has been explored as a less invasive method to achieve high drug concentrations in the vitreous cavity. Periocular administration, where the drug is injected in the vicinity of the ocular organ such as the sub-conjunctival, sub-tenon, and parabulbar regions, is used so that the drug molecules can reach the vitreous cavity by crossing the sclera, choroid, and RPE barriers.[10] Although the risks are lower, this route of delivery is also associated with serious adverse effects such as rise in intraocular pressure (IOP), cataract development, hyphema, strabismus, and corneal decompensation.[11]

Overall, these challenges have hindered the use of many promising therapeutic agents, emphasizing the urgent need to develop novel drug delivery strategies for the eyes. Among various approaches for optimizing drug delivery to the eyes, nanomedicine, particularly the use of nanoparticle-based drug delivery systems, can play an essential role.

Nanomedicine, which exploits nanotechnology to solve medical challenges, has offered numerous exciting possibilities in advancing healthcare. In particular, nanoparticle drugs have become validated therapeutics by formulating nanometer-scale carriers composed of various therapeutic entities, including small-molecule drugs, peptides, proteins and nucleic acids, and excipient materials such as lipids and polymers.[12,13] Although nanoparticle therapeutics were initially developed for cancer treatment, their application has expanded into ophthalmology, owing largely to their unique capability of enhancing drug efficacy through improved drug encapsulation, sustained or triggered drug release, and preferential targeting to disease sites. A few nanoparticle therapeutics have been clinically approved for treating ophthalmic diseases. For example, pegaptanib, an anti-VEGF aptamer conjugated with branched polyethylene glycol, has been applied for the treatment of age-related macular degeneration (AMD).[14]

In addition, nanomedicine has provided new opportunities for overcoming obstacles in treating ophthalmic diseases. For example, the combination of synthetic chemistry with a basic understanding of protein–polymer interactions has led to the efficient encapsulation of proteins within nanoparticles and the controlled delivery of these particles within biological fluid under mild conditions.[15] These technologies are particularly promising, as the therapeutic potential of proteins and monoclonal antibodies is increasingly being realized in ophthalmology, particularly for halting retinal angiogenesis.[16] Nanotechnology has also resulted in the formation of sophisticated carriers that are capable of delivering therapeutic agents to the cytoplasm for bioactivity.[17] Technology for intracellular delivery, if available, can be used in siRNA-based therapeutics to selectively silence gene expression for the treatment of ophthalmic diseases.

Nanomedicine has also provided new opportunities for attaining prolonged ocular drug retention. In particular, approaches that are under active investigation include the incorporation of bioadhesive components to formulate multifunctional nanoparticle drug reservoirs that can be attached to the corneal tissue with high affinity.[18] Furthermore, the recent development of polymeric nanoparticles that are camouflaged by the red blood cell membrane allows man-made delivery vehicles to share functionalities that have been made and perfected by nature, hence taking another step towards bridging synthetic materials with natural components.[19,20] These biomimetic nanoparticles, which have excellent biocompatibility and well-controlled drug release kinetics, will have many applications in the treatment of ophthalmic diseases.

In this chapter, four major nanoparticle platforms for ocular drug delivery are discussed, including liposomes, polymeric nanoparticles, dendrimers, and novel inorganic nanoparticles (Fig. 1). We highlight the unique strengths of each platform and review their recent progress in advancing drug delivery for treating eye diseases.

2. Liposomes

Liposomes are a class of well-established drug delivery platforms.[21,22] A large selection of biocompatible lipids is readily available for formulating liposomes with precisely tailored chemical, biological, and mechanical properties. Owing to their unique self-closed structures, liposomes can entrap hydrophilic agents in their aqueous compartment and hydrophobic agents in the membrane. Structural similarity is also drawn between liposomes and the tear film, providing this class of carriers with excellent ocular biocompatibility. Liposomes protect the loaded drug molecules from external degradation, and their similarity to biological membranes provides unique opportunities to deliver drug molecules into cells and sub-cellular compartments. In addition, various physicochemical properties of liposomes including their size, charge, and surface functional ligands can be altered at different stages of the formulation process, resulting in functionalities favoring different drug delivery tasks. These advantages, collectively, have made liposomes a leading drug delivery

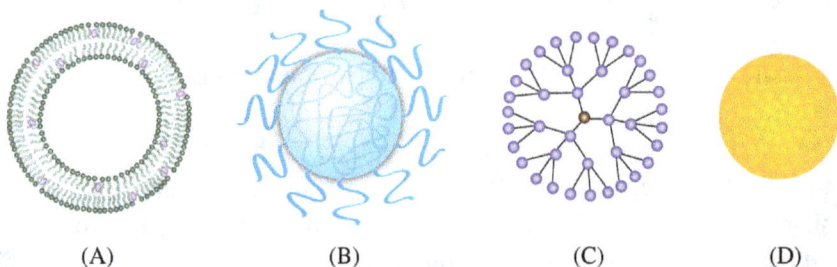

(A)   (B)   (C)   (D)

Figure 1.   Major nanoparticle-based ocular delivery platforms: (A) liposome, (B) polymeric nanoparticle, (C) dendrimer, and (D) inorganic nanoparticle.

platform benefitting a wide range of clinical settings that include various ocular diseases.[23,24]

Liposomes can be topically delivered to the eye surface. In this route, the surface charge strongly affects the interactions between liposomes and the corneal tissues. The mucous membrane of the corneal surface is rich in negatively charged sialic acid moieties. Therefore, when compared with neutral or negatively charged liposomes, those with a positive charge interact strongly with the negatively charged corneal surface, resulting in enhanced corneal retention, reduced drug elimination by lacrymal flow, and enhanced transcorneal flux. In addition, cationic liposomes have been shown to exert adjuvant immunity when they are used for vaccine delivery. For example, cationic liposomes containing the secretory form of herpes simplex virus type 1 (HSV-1), glycoprotein B (gB1s) or two related polylysine-rich peptides, namely DTK1 and DTK2, were investigated for immunotherapeutic potential against HSV-1 infection.[25] The liposomal formulation was able to induce significant protection against lethal ocular challenge. Besides surface charge, liposome rigidity also affects its transport from eye surface to the posterior segment. For example, liposomes made from 1,2-distearoyl-sn-glycero-3-phosphocholine (DSPC) are more rigid than those made from L-α-phosphatidylcholine (egg PC).[26] When administered as eye drops, DSPC liposomes showed a higher accumulation in the retina compared to egg PC liposomes.[27]

The applications of liposomes are frequently limited by their intrinsic instability. Conventional liposomes, particularly with sub-100 nm size, have high surface curvature and are prone to fusing with each other when they collide to minimize their surface tension.[28,29] Such inter-liposome fusion often leads to payload loss or undesired mixing. One strategy to overcome this drawback is to first formulate anionic liposomes, and then coat the liposomes with cationic polymers through electrostatic interactions. The adsorbed polymers not only reverse liposome surface charge from negative to positive, but also act as stabilizers that prevent liposome fusion. In this respect, chitosan, a naturally derived cationic polymer, has gained significant attention.[30–32] Chitosan has been widely explored to modify liposomes for ocular drug delivery. For example, low molecular weight chitosan was readily adsorbed onto the surface of anionic liposomes and thus improved the stability of the liposomes over a 30-day storage period.[33] Chitosan-coated liposomes also showed significantly prolonged precorneal retention and transcorneal penetration in rabbits compared with non-coated liposomes or free drug solution (Fig. 2).[34,35] In another example, chitosan was used to coat liposomes that encapsulated coenzyme Q10 to improve ophthalmic drug delivery.[36] Chitosan improved the permeability of liposomes across the corneal epithelium and delivery of the encapsulated coenzyme Q10, which elevated cell viability under oxidative stress. A similar strategy was also applied to facilitate the

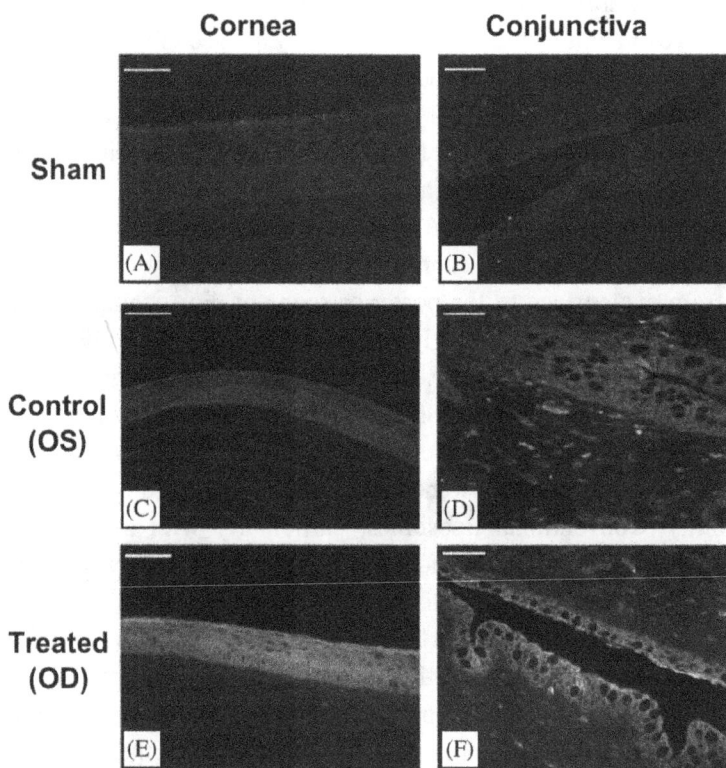

Figure 2. Fluorescence microscopy of rabbit corneal and conjunctival tissue sections. Liposomes were encapsulated with FITC-albumin for fluorescence detection. Tissues were taken 24 h after the initial instillation. Tissues from sham animals (A, B) and control eyes (OS) (C, D) showed no fluorescence while experimental eyes (OD) treated with chitosan-modified liposomes showed fluorescence. Scale bar, 10 μm in (A) and 50 μm in (B–F). Reproduced with permission from Ref. [35].

ocular permeation and delivery of ciprofloxacin-loaded liposomes, leading to enhanced antimicrobial activity of ciprofloxacin against *Pseudomonas aeruginosa* in rabbits' eyes.[37] Besides chitosan, other cationic polymers such as poly-L-lysine (PLL) and polyethylenimine (PEI) can also enhance the delivery of liposomal drugs to retina segments after eye drop administration.[38,39] Taken together, these studies suggest that modifying liposomes with cationic polymers represents an effective strategy to improve transcorneal delivery of liposomal drugs.

Dispersing liposomes into a hydrogel is another novel strategy to improve drug availability for treatment of ocular diseases. For example, liposomes loaded with ofloxacin were first dispersed into a solution of chitosan and β-glycerophosphate, which forms a hydrogel network when elevated to physiological temperature.[40] This liposome-loaded, thermosensitive hydrogel ensures steady, prolonged drug release and higher transcorneal permeation of ofloxacin. A similar strategy can also be applied to make disposable contact lenses as vehicles for ophthalmic drug delivery.[41]

In addition to topical delivery, drug-loaded liposomes can be administered through intravitreal injection for prolonged drug release to the posterior segment of the eyes. In this case, polymers are commonly used to coat liposomes for enhanced stability.[42] For example, polyethylene glycol (PEG) coated liposomes were loaded with short oligothymidylate and then injected into the vitreous.[43] Compared to free drug, the liposomal formulation provided sustained release of oligothymidylate and resulted in better accumulation of drug molecules at the retina-choroid region.

Niosomes are a special type of liposome, which are prepared from uncharged single-chain surfactant and cholesterol.[44] Although niosomes share many characteristics with conventional liposomes, they are considered to have better chemical stability and lower cost for manufacturing.[45] Similar to liposomes, niosomes are efficient carriers for small hydrophilic molecules such as naltrexone, acetazolamide and gentamicin, and they provide improved corneal retention and prolonged release. Mixing niosomes with mucoadhesive polymers such as chitosan and Carbopol® in suspension can further prolong therapeutic efficacy while reducing systemic absorption.[46]

Recently, monoolein, a molecule composed of a hydrocarbon chain attached to a glycerol through an ester bond, has been shown to have mucoadhesive properties desirable for eye delivery.[47,48] It is intriguing that monoolein can form cubic nanoparticles, named cubosomes, and these particles do not induce any obvious ocular irritation. The amphiphilic nature of monoolein allows cubosomes to load a wide range of drug molecules. For example, monoolein cubosomes loaded with dexamethasone significantly improved preocular retention, ocular bioavailability, and the apparent permeability of the drug molecules. The therapeutic potential of monoolein cubosomes was also demonstrated in the delivery of flurbiprofen and cyclosporine A, where cubosomes significantly enhanced the transcorneal permeation of both drugs.[47,48]

3. Polymeric Nanoparticles

Polymeric nanoparticles offer a variety of advantages and have a wide array of applications in the field of drug delivery.[49,50] They are commonly formulated through the self-assembly of amphiphilic block copolymers, of which the hydrophilic block forms a shell while the hydrophobic block forms a core. During the nanoparticle preparation process via a nanoprecipitation, emulsion or solvent replacement technique, therapeutic agents ranging from small hydrophobic molecules to large hydrophilic agents such as proteins and nucleic acids can be encapsulated within the particles. Numerous biodegradable and biocompatible polymers with established safety profiles are available for nanoparticle formulations, resulting in several robust platforms with significant potential for translation.[14] These include poly(lactic-co-glycolic acid) (PLGA), poly(lactic acid) (PLA), and polycaprolactone (PCL), all of which have validated applications in the clinic. With these benefits, polymeric nanoparticle-based drug delivery has shown significant promise in the treatment of various ocular diseases.[51]

Nanoparticle encapsulation enhances drug solubility and provides sustained and controlled release. A large number of drug molecules with poor water solubility such as sparfloxacin, levofloxacin, acyclovir, celecoxib, and cyclosporine have been successfully encapsulated into polymeric nanoparticles for ocular delivery.[52–54] Compared to free drug molecules, nanoparticles allow the drug molecules to be confined within the ocular region (Fig. 3). The release kinetics are determined by both drug diffusion from the nanoparticles and hydrolytic erosion of the polymers. Polymeric

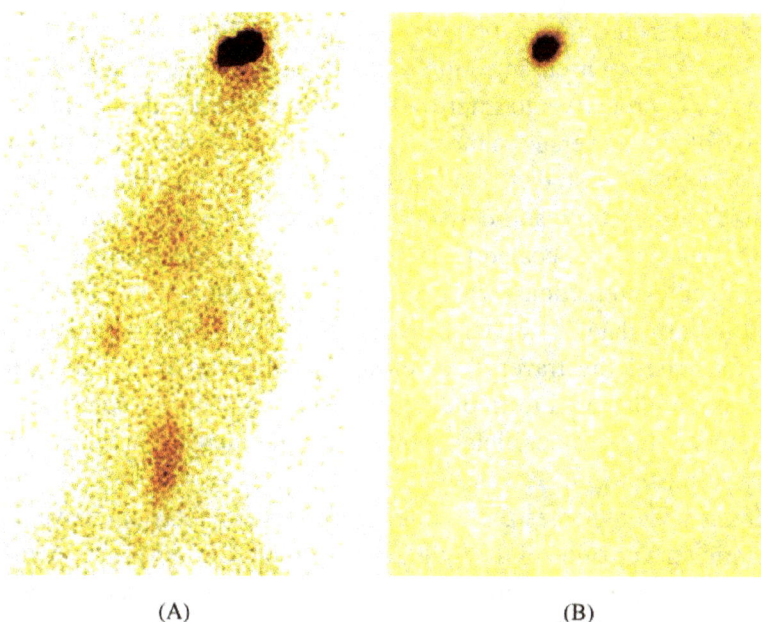

(A)   (B)

Figure 3. Gamma scintigraphic static whole body images 5 h after administration of (A) a marketed formulation of levofloxacin, and (B) levofloxacin-loaded PLGA nanoparticles. Levofloxacin was radiolabeled with Tc-99 m by using stannous chloride as the reducing agent. The radiolabeled drug molecules were encapsulated into PLGA nanoparticles through nanoprecipitation. 50 μL of the radiolabeled formulation was instilled onto the left corneal surface of each rabbit. The images were taken 5 h after the initial instillation. Reproduced with permission from Ref. [52].

nanoparticles have also attracted much attention for gene delivery to treat ocular diseases. In particular, plasmids expressing antiangiogenic proteins such as plasminogen kringle 5 and VEGF-A inhibitor have been delivered using PLGA nanoparticles with some success in treating choroidal neo-vascularization and retinal inflammation.[55] In addition, PLGA nanoparticles have been used to encapsulate siRNA molecules with the potential to modulate angiogenesis and vascular function through interfering gene expression in primary endothelial cells.[2]

The surface coating of polymeric nanoparticles plays a significant role in determining the pharmacokinetics of the nanoparticles *in vivo*. For systemic delivery through intravenous injection, PEG has become the gold standard for nanoparticle surface coating. However, for topical delivery or intravitreal injection to the eyes, other materials have shown compelling properties to improve therapeutic efficacy. For example, the effect of PEG versus chitosan surface modification on polymeric nanoparticles was studied and the two polymer coatings showed differing abilities to penetrate and deliver drug molecules across the corneal tissue.[56] Chitosan was coated to the surface of PCL nanoparticles through electrostatic interactions, whereas the block copolymer PCL-b-PEG was used to formulate PEG-coated nanoparticles. Although both nanoparticles increased the traversal of encapsulated drugs across the corneal epithelium compared to free drug molecules, at 4 h post-administration, chitosan-coated nanoparticles showed a 3-fold increase in the amount of drug permeation.

It has been hypothesized that nanoparticles may play an active role in enlarging the opening of the tight junction of ocular tissues and increasing the use of paracellular pathways for drug penetration.[57] As a result, various types of amphiphilic copolymers with unique surface coatings have demonstrated their ability to improve the *in vivo* bioavailability of the encapsulated drugs. For example, the triblock copolymer poly(ethylene oxide)-*block*-poly(propylene oxide)-*block*-poly(ethylene oxide) (PEO-PPO-PEO) was used to formulate nanoparticles, where the hydrophobic PPO core is surrounded by an outer shell of hydrated PEO. Nanoparticles loaded with pilocarpine showed a 64% increase in miotic response compared to a standard pilocarpine eye-drop solution.[58] Nanoparticles formulated with the same PEO-PPO-PEO triblock copolymer were also found to increase the stability and penetration of DNA plasmids when applied to corneal tissues. In addition, the correlation among PEO-PPO-PEO triblock composition, micellar structure, and salt-in-polymer solubility was investigated, suggesting that this triblock polymer could efficiently encapsulate various hydrophobic drug molecules for ocular delivery.[59]

Polymeric nanoparticles that form stable suspensions in aqueous environments have also been widely used to improve ocular drug bioavailability through intravitreal injection.[60] For example, antisense oligonucleotides were encapsulated in polymeric nanoparticles made from poly(ethylene oxide)-*block*-polyspermine (PEO-*b*-PSP).[61] Following intravitreal injection of the nanoparticles into rats, fluorescently labeled oligonucleotides were detected in retinal vascular cells at 24 h post-injection and persisted for 6 days, the endpoint of this study. The nanoparticles successfully reduced the expression of fibronectin mRNA levels to 86.7% two days after injection and to 46.7% on day 6. In another study, nanoparticles were formulated with chitosan-carbohydrate amphiphilic copolymers and showed significantly improved capacity in loading prednisolone compared to that of pluronic block copolymers.[62] Upon both intravitreal injection and topical ocular application of the nanoparticles, the bioavailability of prednisolone had a 10-fold increase compared to a commercial emulsion formulation of the same drug.

Polymeric nanoparticles responsive to environmental cues for triggered drug release have also been explored for ocular drug delivery. For example, a triblock copolymer comprising N-isopropylacrylamide (NIPAAM), vinylpyrrolidone (VP), and acrylic acid (AA) was cross-linked with N, N-methylenebis(acrylamide) (MBA) to form nanoparticles that could efficiently load drug molecules at ambient temperature (25°C) and provide fast release at physiological temperature (37°C).[63] The nanoparticles were investigated for the delivery of ketorolac tromethamine, an anti-inflammatory drug. *In vitro* corneal permeation studies through excised rabbit cornea showed a 2-fold increase in ocular availability with no corneal damage compared to an aqueous suspension containing the same amount of drug as in the nanoparticle formulation. The formulation showed significant inhibition of lid closure up to 3 h and PMN migration up to 5 h while the suspension containing non-entrapped drug did not show any significant effect.

4. Dendrimers

Dendrimers are a class of macromolecules with a branched structure around a central core.[64] They are liquid or semi-solid polymers commonly decorated with amine, carboxylic or hydroxyl surface groups. Dendrimers have a high density of surface functional groups, which allows them to interact strongly with corneal tissues. In particular, for amine-terminated dendrimers, a larger fraction of the surface amine groups protonates at pathological pH values (pH = 5.5 for tear fluid), which favors dendrimer binding with ocular mucins.[65] This strong interaction in turn increases the retention time and the permeation of dendrimers, resulting in enhanced drug availability across the corneal layers. Intriguingly, even dendrimers with negatively charged surface carboxylic groups show mucoadhesive properties.[66] These anionic dendrimers are found to interact strongly with the nonglycosylated domains of the mucins, which possess positively charged amino acid residues. Owing to their unique structures and corneal binding properties, dendrimers have been extensively explored for ocular drug delivery.[67]

Among various dendrimer molecules, polyamidoamine (PAMAM)-based dendrimers have received the most attention. For example, they have been explored as combination therapy for preventing scar tissue formation and improving the long-term success of glaucoma infiltration surgery.[68] Specifically, PAMAM dendrimers were conjugated with glucosamine, which prevented the activation and maturation of dendritic cells by suppressing the LPS-activated TLR-4 pathway. Meanwhile, some dendrimers were conjugated with glucosamine-6-sulfate, which inhibits endothelial cell proliferation by blocking the fibroblast growth factor-2, thereby preventing microtubule formation and neoangiogenesis. Through subconjunctival administration, this combinatorial dendrimer system inhibited scar tissue formation and increased the long-term success rate from 30% to 80% in rabbit models of glaucoma infiltration surgery without inducing tissue inflammation and infection (Fig. 4).

Dendrimers showed a significantly lower ocular irritation index compared with Carbopol-solutions.[69] For treating open-angle glaucoma, PAMAM dendrimers were also used to deliver pilocarpine and tropicamide, two effective drugs suffering from poor permeability and low stability.[70] Dendrimer formulations were more efficacious compared with commercially available Carbopol-eye drop formulations and showed no disturbance in visual acuity when instilled on the corneal surface. Phosphorous dendrimers were also developed as a stabilizer for carteolol, an antihypertensive drug used to treat glaucoma, as the traditional preservative benzalkonium chloride is toxic and damages the protective barriers in the cornea. Topically instilled dendrimer-carteolol conjugate solutions produced no irritation even after several hours in rabbit corneas and showed increased precorneal residence time compared to PAMAM–COOH dendrimers. Moreover, the quantity of carteolol in the aqueous humor was

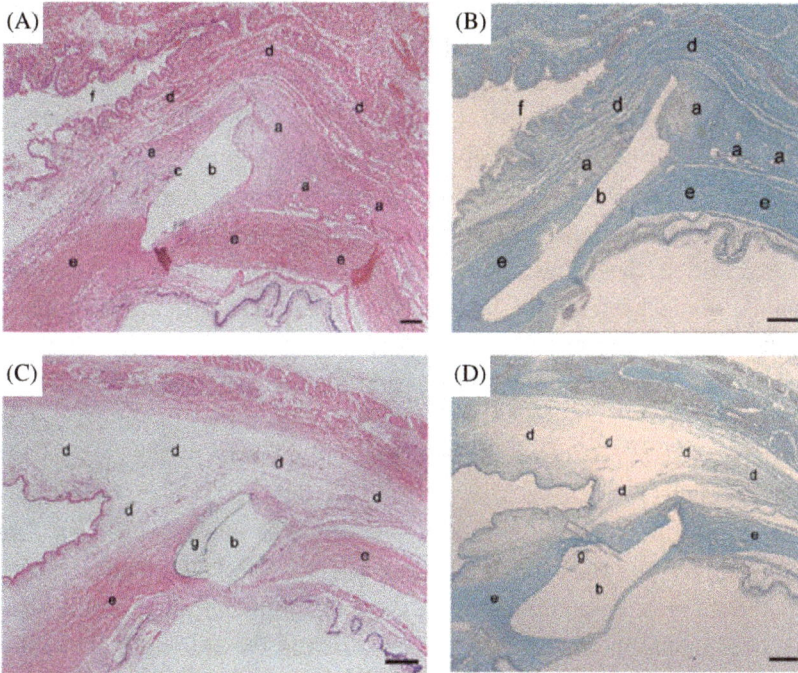

Figure 4. Polyvalent PAMAM dendrimer-glucosamine conjugates prevent scar tissue formation. (A, B) Histological cross-sections stained with hematoxylin & eosin and Masson's trichrome, respectively, from a control rabbit eye at day 30 after surgery. Masson's trichrome stains collagen green and muscle red. The sections show that the surgical drainage channel is surrounded by hypercellular scar tissue containing collagen. This extensive scar tissue formation prevents the drainage of the aqueous humor across the conjunctiva and leads to the failure of the surgery. (C, D) Histological cross-sections stained with hematoxylin & eosin and Masson's trichrome, respectively, from a dendrimer glucosamine treated rabbit eye at day 30 after surgery. The sections show that the surgical drainage channel and cannula are surrounded by loose connective tissue. There is minimal scar tissue formation. This means that the aqueous humor can drain across the conjunctiva and that the surgery has been successful. Normal collagen fibrils are seen in the cornea in all sections. a, scar tissue; b, channel; c, stitch material; d, conjunctiva; e, cornea; f, fornix; g, cannula. Scale bars, 1 mm. Reproduced with permission from Ref. [68].

~2.5-fold higher when compared to animals treated with carteolol solutions, suggesting improved bioavailability. As another example, PAMAM (G3-NH$_2$) dendrimers stabilized with surface conjugated PEG chains were used to load hydrophobic antiglaucomatic agents such as brimonidine and timolol maleate into their hydrophobic cores to increase the bioavailability of these drugs after topical instillation.[71,72] Through the terminal acrylate groups on the PEG chains, these dendrimers cross-linked to form a water-soluble viscous solution upon UV irradiation. Such a dendrimer formulation possessed better mucoadhesive properties due to a large number of surface anionic groups, sustained release with no cytotoxic effects, and enhanced corneal transport of the loaded drug molecules.

In addition, dendrimers have been explored for antimicrobial treatment against corneal infections. In fact, dendrimer nanoparticles alone can be used as topical antimicrobial agents. For example, PAMAM dendrimers showed bactericidal activity against gram-negative bacteria such as *E. coli* to treat chorioamnionitis.[73] The antibacterial mechanism seems dependent on the surface functional groups of the dendrimer. PAMAM G4-NH_2 dendrimers act as polycations that can actively interact with the bacterial cell wall, compromising the cell wall integrity and causing bacteria death. Interestingly, anionic dendrimers such as G4-COOH also showed antibacterial activities by chelating the positive calcium and magnesium ions of the cell membrane and therefore destabilizing the cell wall. Dendrimers can also be used as delivery vehicles for antibiotics against corneal infection.[74,75] For example, PAMAM dendrimers were shown to enhance the solubility of hydrophobic quinolones such as nadifloxacin and prulifloxacin.[76] As a class of dendrimers with triolyl branches and surface guanidine groups, dendrimeric polyguanidilyated translocators (DPTs) showed potential as ophthalmic carriers for gatifloxacin (GFX), a fourth generation fluoroquinolone approved for the treatment of conjunctivitis. Other novel classes of dendrimers, such as glycodendrimers, polypropylenimine, anionic amphiphilic dendrimers, polylysine dendrimers, and oligosaccharide dendrimers, have also been explored either alone as antibacterial agents or as delivery vehicles for antimicrobial drugs that treating a variety of corneal, conjunctival, and intraocular infections.

Dendrimers have also been used as potential ocular sealants for accelerating corneal wound healing. The cornea is a transparent tissue devoid of blood vessels and possesses highly ordered stromal collagen fibrils critical for clear vision. Wounds caused by trauma, surgeries, and corneal transplantation require sutures to fasten the corneal flaps, which sometimes imposes a high risk of perturbing normal vision. A new class of dendrimers with compatible biopolymers was developed for photo-curable corneal adhesion.[77] These dendrimers can form transparent layers that not only rapidly seal the corneal lacerations, but also act as temporary scaffolds for corneal regeneration.[78] The dendrimer sealant also avoided the irregular healing, inflammation, and scar tissue formation commonly seen on sutured cornea.[79]

Furthermore, dendrimers have been extensively explored to treat intraocular posterior segment diseases. For example, PAMAM loaded with fluocinolone acetonide was used for the attenuation of activated microglia.[80] These dendrimer-drug conjugates exhibited sustained release of fluocinolone acetonide for three months, thereby offering the potential to enhance the bioavailability of the drug to the target cells in the retina for an extended period of time. Upon intravitreal administration, the conjugates were found to preferentially accumulate in activated microglia and photoreceptors, and were present in the microglial cells even after 30 days post-injection. Interestingly, a single intravitreal injection showed significant attenuation of activated microglial cells at a 30-fold lower dosage compared to free drug, with no cytotoxic effect. Electroretinography experiments showed favorable preservation of photoreceptor function, indicating neuroprotection activity in RCS rat models. In another example, a novel class of peptide dendrimers containing SB105 and SB105 A10 peptides as building blocks built on a biocompatible lysine core was recently developed. These dendrimers inhibited several viral strains by blocking the heparin sulfate polysaccharides critical for viral entry. In addition, PAMAM dendrimers with carboxyl surface groups were used to load carboplatin to treat intraocular tumors.[81] Encapsulation of chemo-therapeutic drug molecules into the dendrimers effectively extended the half-life of the drug molecules while decreasing their toxicity. Dendrimers can also be conjugated with surface ligands for ocular tumor targeting. For example, dendrimers comprised of prophyrin-based glycopolymers bound strongly to the surface lectins of ocular tumors.[82] They were then conjugated with Concanavalin A, a mannose-specific ligand protein, that further enhanced targeting specificity to tumor cells in the retina. This dual-targeting dendrimer platform was applied as a photosensitizer for preferential accumulation in malignant ocular tissue to enhance photodynamic therapy.

Cationic dendrimers have also attracted much attention for gene and siRNA delivery.[83] Polycationic dendrimers can complex with siRNA molecules, protect them from degradation, and facilitate endosomal escape for bioactivity. Dendrimers can be also conjugated with cell-penetrating peptides for efficient endosomal escape.[84] Dendrimer-based photosensitizers using phthalocyanine as material for the particle cores can be used to compact therapeutic genes with a targeting approach mediated by irradiation.[85] Upon subconjunctival injection of the above dendrimer formulation followed by laser irradiation, transgene expression was observed only in the irradiated areas. Such strategies may be useful in the case of macular degeneration where neuroprotective genes can be administered intravitreally, and directed only to the macular area via photoillumination.

5. Inorganic Nanoparticles

Owing to their unique anatomical and physiological characteristics, eyes are isolated from the rest of the body by various barriers. Although these barriers restrict the bioavailability of drug molecules delivered to the eyes, they also minimize their systemic exposure and potentially reduce toxicity concerns. As a result, various inorganic nanoparticles that are otherwise suboptimal for systemic treatment can become useful for treating ocular diseases.[86] Among various inorganic nanoparticles, gold nanoparticles have found widespread applications as drug carriers and imaging agents in biology and medicine as a result of their biocompatibility, optical properties, and easily modifiable surfaces.[87,88] They have also been explored for treating various ocular diseases.

Intriguingly, various inorganic nanoparticles have been found to be efficacious agents for the treatment of pathological angiogenesis. Pathological angiogenesis in the retina is the major cause of vision loss at all ages. In particular, retinopathy of prematurity (ROP) is a leading cause of blindness in children. Studies found that intravitreal injection of gold nanoparticles with a diameter of 20 nm inhibited retinal neovascularization in a mouse model of ROP (Fig. 5).[89] In addition, gold nanoparticles effectively suppressed signs of vascular endothelial growth factor (VEGF)-induced angiogenesis of retinal microvascular endothelial cells *in vitro* including proliferation, migration and capillary-like network

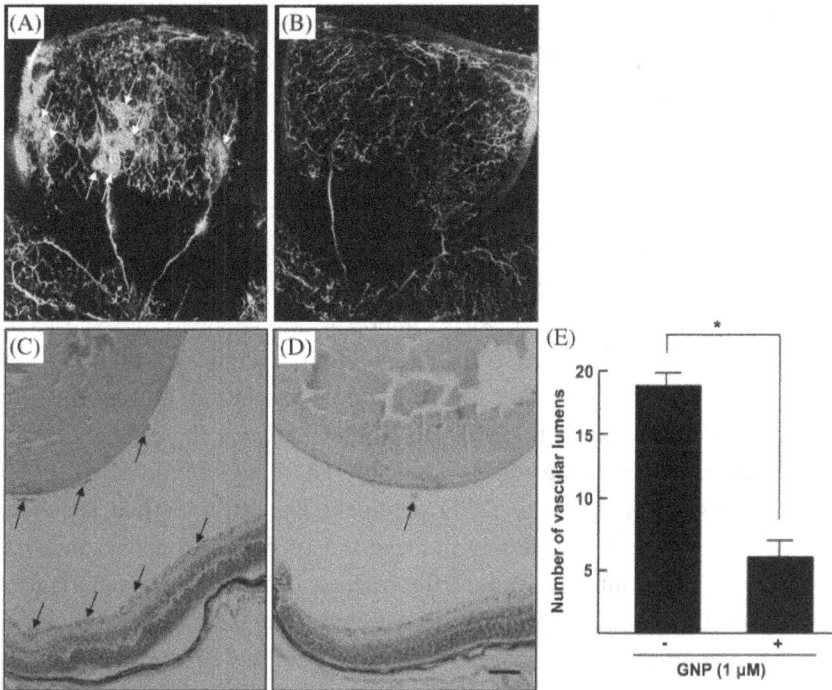

Figure 5. Inhibition of retinal neovascularization in mice with oxygen-induced retino-pathy (OIR) by gold nanoparticles (20 nm diameter). The pups were injected intravi-treously with 1 μM gold nanoparticle solution on postnatal day (P) 14, when retinal neovascularization began. At P 17, the eyes were removed for analysis. (A, B) Retinal vasculature in control and nanoparticle injected mice with OIR was evaluated by fluores-cein angiography using fluorescein conjugated dextran. Arrows indicate neovascular tufts of intravitreous neovascularization. (C, D) Hematoxylin-stained cross-sections prepared from control (C) and gold nanoparticle-injected (D) mice, respectively. Arrows indicate the vascular lumens of new vessels growing into the vitreous cavity. Scale bars: 100 μm. (E) Each value represents the mean ± SD of three independent experiments. *$p < 0.05$. Reproduced with permission from Ref. [89].

formation. Gold nanoparticles also blocked VEGF-induced autophos-phorylation of VEGFR-2, which consequently inhibited EFK 1/2 acti-vation. The intrinsic antiangiogenic property of gold nanoparticles was also applied to treat proliferative vitreo-retinopathy (PVR), one of the major ocular complications after retinal injury or retinal detachment surgery.[90] Although various growth factors are elevated during PVR, a VEGF-induced signaling network and the chemotactic effect of inter-leukin-1 beta (IL-1β) are considered major factors that stimulate the proliferation and migration of RPE cells. Following intravitreal injection, gold nanoparticles with a diameter of 50 nm binds to the heparin binding domains of VEGF165, most likely through the reactive thiol groups, and blocks the VEGF- and IL-1β-dependent cell spreading, migration, and proliferation in bovine RPE cells.

Meanwhile, other inorganic nanoparticles have also been found to be antiangiogenic. For example, silver nanoparticles can also inhibit VEGF-induced retinal endothelial cells; the inhibitory activities of the nanoparticles were shown to result from down-regulation of the Src and AKT/PI3K signaling pathways.[91] To further enhance the efficacy, silver nanoparticles were encapsulated with poly(gamma glutamic acid) (PGA) and conjugated with cyclic RGD peptides. The particles had sustained release of PGA and specifically induced the apoptosis of neovascularization cells.[92] The antiangiogenic effect against retinal neovascularization was also demonstrated with silicate nanoparticles.[93] No direct toxicity of these nanoparticles was observed on retinal neuronal or endothelial cells, nor was it observed on the retinal tissue. Furthermore, intravitreal injection of silicate nanoparticles reduced anomalous retinal angiogenesis in oxygen-induced retinopathy mice. They also effectively inhibited VEGF-induced angiogenesis *in vitro*. Via suppression of VEGF receptor-2 phosphorylation induced by VEGF, silicate nanoparticles were able to block ERK 1/2 activation. Taken together, these studies suggest that inorganic nanoparticles may become useful as safe inhibitors for retinal neovascularization.

Besides their use as a direct anti-angiogenesis agent, gold nanoparticles have also been used as enhancers for radiotherapy. For AMD, photodynamic therapy and antiangiogenic pharmacotherapy represent the standard of care for most patients. However, these therapies require repeated treatments or injections, putting the patient at risk for cataract formation, endophthalmitis, vitreous hemorrhage, and retinal detachment in addition to creating logistical difficulties and patient discomfort. Recently, the dosimetric feasibility of using gold nanoparticles as radiosensitizers to enhance kilovoltage stereotactic radiosurgery for neovascular AMD was theoretically evaluated.[94] The analysis showed that dose enhancement was markedly confined to the targeted neovascular AMD endothelial cells where the nanoparticles were localized. The findings provided an impetus for considering the application of gold nanoparticles to enhance therapeutic efficacy during stereotactic radiosurgery for neovascular AMD.

Various neurodegenerative diseases are known to occur and progress because of oxidative stress, which results from the presence of reactive oxygen species (ROS) in excess of what can be handled naturally by cells. In this respect, cerium oxide nanoparticles (nanoceria), which have been shown to have minimal cytotoxicity to ocular tissues, can catalytically scavenge ROS by mimicking the activities of superoxide dismutase and catalase.[95] A single intravitreal injection of nanoceria into a Vldlr-/- eye was shown to inhibit the rise of ROS in the Vldlr-/- retina, the increase of VEGF in the photoreceptor layer, and the formation of intraretinal and subretinal neovascular lesions.[96] Of more therapeutic interest, injection of nanoceria into older mice (postnatal day 28) resulted in the regression of existing vascular lesions, indicating that pathological neovessels require the continual production of excessive ROS. The results demonstrated the unique ability of nanoceria to prevent downstream effects of oxidative stress, indicating great therapeutic potential for the treatment of neurodegenerative diseases such as AMD and diabetic retinopathy.

The majority of treatment modalities for glaucoma so far have been focused on dropping intraocular pressure (IOP) by drug administration or surgical operation. These methods have been found to temporarily cure glaucoma, however there has been no efficacious modality to completely treat glaucoma as well as to protect optic nerves from glaucoma-induced mechanical damage. The induction of heat shock proteins (HSPs) has been recently considered to be a new powerful modality for the protection of optic nerves from glaucoma. However, the current clinical approaches to inducing HSPs in retinal ganglion cells (RGCs) are limited due to undesirable side effects. Recently, engineered superparamagnetic $Mn_{0.5}Zn_{0.5}Fe_2O_4$ nanoparticles (EMZF-SPNPAs) with a 5.5 nm mean particle size were explored to induce HSPs through local magnetic hyperthermia. These nanoparticles were considered a promising localized HSP-induction agent because of their unique features, which include sufficiently high specific absorption rate (SAR) achieved within a biologically safe range of applied AC magnetic field and frequency as well as superior biocompatibility. The study also demonstrated a novel infusion technique in which the EMZF-SPNPAs were able to diffuse through the vitreous body to the retina in a rat eye. Overall, the technique is promising as a safe ocular neuroprotection modality.

6. Outlook

The advent of nanotechnology, together with the accumulation of knowledge on ocular diseases, has enabled significant advancement in the field of ophthalmologic drug delivery. As reviewed in this chapter, efforts have been given to various nanoparticle-based drug delivery platforms which include liposomes, polymeric nanoparticles, dendrimers, and inorganic nanoparticles. These advanced nanoparticle delivery systems have effectively improved ocular drug bioavailability and offered valuable opportunities in creating novel therapeutic paradigms such as intracellular delivery and combinatorial therapy. The advancement of nanotechnology will allow for continuing improvement of ocular drug delivery systems with the aim of achieving more efficacious, patient-compliant, and cost-effective therapeutics for the treatment of various ocular diseases.

7. References

1. Zhang, K., Zhang, L. & Weinreb, R.N. Ophthalmic drug discovery: Novel targets and mechanisms for retinal diseases and glaucoma. *Nat Rev Drug Discovery* **11**, 541–559 (2012).
2. Gaudana, R., Jwala, J., Boddu, S.H.S. & Mitra, A.K. Recent perspectives in ocular drug delivery. *Pharm Res* **26**, 1197–1216 (2009).
3. Hughes, P.M., Olejnik, O., Chang-Lin, J.E. & Wilson, C.G. Topical and systemic drug delivery to the posterior segments. *Adv Drug Delivery Rev* **57**, 2010–2032 (2005).
4. Peng, C.C., *et al.* Emulsions and microemulsions for ocular drug delivery. *J Drug Del Sci Tech* **21**, 111–121 (2011).
5. del Amo, E.M. & Urtti, A. Current and future ophthalmic drug delivery systems. A shift to the posterior segment. *Drug Discov Today* **13**, 135–143 (2008).

6. Yasukawa, T., *et al.* Drug delivery systems for vitreoretinal diseases. *Prog Retin Eye Res* **23**, 253–281 (2004).

7. Kolomeyer, A.M., Roy, M.S. & Chu, D.S. The use of intravitreal ranibizumab for choroidal neovascularization associated with vogt-koyanagi-harada syndrome. *Case Rep Med* **2011**, 747648–747648 (2011).

8. Harder, B.C., von Baltz, S., Jonas, J.B. & Schlichtenbrede, F.C. Intravitreal bevacizumab for retinopathy of prematurity. *J Ocul Pharmacol Ther* **27**, 623–627 (2011).

9. Harder, B.C., *et al.* Intravitreal bevacizumab for retinopathy of prematurity: Refractive error results. *Am J Ophthalmol* **155**, 1119–1124 (2013).

10. Hao, J., Yang, M.B., Liu, H. & Li, S.K. Distribution of propranolol in periocular tissues: A comparison of topical and systemic administration. *J Ocul Pharmacol Ther* **27**, 453–459 (2011).

11. Ung, T. & Currie, Z.I. Periocular changes following long-term administration of latanoprost 0.005%. *Ophthal Plast Reconstr Surg* **28**, E42–E44 (2012).

12. Petros, R.A. & DeSimone, J.M. Strategies in the design of nanoparticles for therapeutic applications. *Nat Rev Drug Discovery* **9**, 615–627 (2010).

13. Shi, J., Votruba, A.R., Farokhzad, O.C. & Langer, R. Nanotechnology in drug delivery and tissue engineering: From discovery to applications. *Nano Lett* **10**, 3223–3230 (2010).

14. Zhang, L., *et al.* Nanoparticles in medicine: Therapeutic applications and developments. *Clin Pharmacol Ther* **83**, 761–769 (2008).

15. Yan, M., *et al.* A novel intracellular protein delivery platform based on single-protein nanocapsules. *Nat Nanotechnol* **5**, 48–53 (2010).

16. Gariano, R.F. & Gardner, T.W. Retinal angiogenesis in development and disease. *Nature* **438**, 960–966 (2005).

17. Whitehead, K.A., Langer, R. & Anderson, D.G. Knocking down barriers: Advances in sirna delivery. *Nat Rev Drug Discovery* **8**, 129–138 (2009).

18. du Toit, L.C., Pillay, V., Choonara, Y.E., Govender, T. & Carmichael, T. Ocular drug delivery — a look towards nanobioadhesives. *Expert Opin Drug Deliv* **8**, 71–94 (2011).

19. Hu, C.-M.J., *et al.* Erythrocyte membrane-camouflaged polymeric nanoparticles as a biomimetic delivery platform. *Proc Natl Acad Sci USA* **108**, 10980–10985 (2011).

20. Hu, C.-M.J., Fang, R.H., Copp, J., Luk, B.T. & Zhang, L. A biomimetic nanosponge that absorbs pore-forming toxins. *Nat Nanotechnol* **8**, 336–340 (2013).

21. Torchilin, V.P. Recent advances with liposomes as pharmaceutical carriers. *Nat Rev Drug Discovery* **4**, 145–160 (2005).
22. Gao, W., Hu, C.-M.J., Fang, R.H. & Zhang, L. Liposome-like nanostructures for drug delivery. *J Mater Chem B* **1**, 6569–6585 (2013).
23. Honda, M., *et al.* Liposomes and nanotechnology in drug development: Focus on ocular targets. *Int J Nanomedicine* **8**, 495–504 (2013).
24. Gan, L., *et al.* Recent advances in topical ophthalmic drug delivery with lipid-based nanocarriers. *Drug Discov Today* **18**, 290–297 (2013).
25. Cortesi, R., *et al.* Cationic liposomes as potential carriers for ocular administration of peptides with anti-herpetic activity. *Int J Pharm* **317**, 90–100 (2006).
26. Ulrich, A.S. Biophysical aspects of using liposomes as delivery vehicles. *Biosci Rep* **22**, 129–150 (2002).
27. Hironaka, K., *et al.* Design and evaluation of a liposomal delivery system targeting the posterior segment of the eye. *J Control Release* **136**, 247–253 (2009).
28. Lei, G.H. & MacDonald, R.C. Lipid bilayer vesicle fusion: Intermediates captured by high-speed microfluorescence spectroscopy. *Biophys J* **85**, 1585–1599 (2003).
29. Haluska, C.K., *et al.* Time scales of membrane fusion revealed by direct imaging of vesicle fusion with high temporal resolution. *Proc Natl Acad Sci USA* **103**, 15841–15846 (2006).
30. Bernkop-Schnuerch, A. & Duennhaupt, S. Chitosan-based drug delivery systems. *Eur. J Pharm Biopharm* **81**, 463–469 (2012).
31. Hu, L., Sun, Y. & Wu, Y. Advances in chitosan-based drug delivery vehicles. *Nanoscale* **5**, 3103–3111 (2013).
32. Sezer, A.D. & Cevher, E. Topical drug delivery using chitosan nano- and microparticles. *Expert Opin Drug Deliv* **9**, 1129–1146 (2012).
33. Felt, O., *et al.* Topical use of chitosan in ophthalmology: Tolerance assessment and evaluation of precorneal retention. *Int J Pharm* **180**, 185–193 (1999).
34. Paolicelli, P., de la Fuente, M., Sanchez, A., Seijo, B. & Jose Alonso, M. Chitosan nanoparticles for drug delivery to the eye. *Expert Opin Drug Deliv* **6**, 239–253 (2009).
35. Diebold, Y., *et al.* Ocular drug delivery by liposome-chitosan nanoparticle complexes (lcs-np). *Biomaterials* **28**, 1553–1564 (2007).
36. Wang, S., *et al.* Protective effect of coenzyme q(10) against oxidative damage in human lens epithelial cells by novel ocular drug carriers. *Int J Pharm* **403**, 219–229 (2011).

37. Mehanna, M.M., Elmaradny, H.A. & Samaha, M.W. Mucoadhesive liposomes as ocular delivery system: Physical, microbiological, and *in vivo* assessment. *Drug Dev Ind Pharm* **36**, 108–118 (2010).

38. Toropainen, E., Hornof, M., Kaarniranta, K., Johansson, P. & Urtti, A. Corneal epithelium as a platform for secretion of transgene products after transfection with liposomal gene eyedrops. *J Gene Med* **9**, 208–216 (2007).

39. Sasaki, H., *et al.* Retinal drug delivery using eyedrop preparations of poly-l-lysine-modified liposomes. *Eur J Pharm Biopharm* **83**, 364–369 (2013).

40. Hosny, K.M. Preparation and evaluation of thermosensitive liposomal hydrogel for enhanced transcorneal permeation of ofloxacin. *Aaps Pharmscitech* **10**, 1336–1342 (2009).

41. Danion, A., Brochu, H., Martin, Y. & Vermette, P. Fabrication and characterization of contact lenses bearing surface-immobilized layers of intact liposomes. *J Biomed Mater Res, Part A* **82A**, 41–51 (2007).

42. Bochot, A. & Fattal, E. Liposomes for intravitreal drug delivery: A state of the art. *J Control Release* **161**, 628–634 (2012).

43. Bochot, A., *et al.* Intravitreal delivery of oligonucleotides by sterically stabilized liposomes. *Invest Ophthalmol Vis Sci* **43**, 253–259 (2002).

44. Mahale, N.B., Thakkar, P.D., Mali, R.G., Walunj, D.R. & Chaudhari, S.R. Niosomes: Novel sustained release nonionic stable vesicular systems — an overview. *Adv Colloid Interface Sci* **183**, 46–54 (2012).

45. Hamishehkar, H., Rahimpour, Y. & Kouhsoltani, M. Niosomes as a propitious carrier for topical drug delivery. *Expert Opin Drug Deliv* **10**, 261–272 (2013).

46. Aggarwal, D. & Kaur, I.P. Improved pharmacodynamics of timolol maleate from a mucoadhesive niosomal ophthalmic drug delivery system. *Int J Pharm* **290**, 155–159 (2005).

47. Garg, G., Saraf, S. & Saraf, S. Cubosomes: An overview. *Biol Pharm Bull* **30**, 350–353 (2007).

48. Spicer, P.T. Progress in liquid crystalline dispersions: Cubosomes. *Curr Opin Colloid Interface Sci* **10**, 274–279 (2005).

49. Shi, J., Xiao, Z., Kamaly, N. & Farokhzad, O.C. Self-assembled targeted nanoparticles: Evolution of technologies and bench to bedside translation. *Acc Chem Res* **44**, 1123–1134 (2011).

50. Colson, Y.L. & Grinstaff, M.W. Biologically responsive polymeric nanoparticles for drug delivery. *Adv Mater* **24**, 3878–3886 (2012).

51. Nagarwal, R.C., Kant, S., Singh, P.N., Maiti, P. & Pandit, J.K. Polymeric nanoparticulate system: A potential approach for ocular drug delivery. *J Control Release* **136**, 2–13 (2009).

52. Gupta, H., *et al.* Biodegradable levofloxacin nanoparticles for sustained ocular drug delivery. *J Drug Target* **19**, 409–417 (2011).
53. Gupta, H., *et al.* Sparfloxacin-loaded plga nanoparticles for sustained ocular drug delivery. *Nanomed-Nanotechn Biol Med* **6**, 324–333 (2010).
54. Li, R., *et al.* A potential new therapeutic system for glaucoma: Solid lipid nanoparticles containing methazolamide. *J Microencapsul* **28**, 134–141 (2011).
55. Park, K., *et al.* Nanoparticle-mediated expression of an angiogenic inhibitor ameliorates ischemia-induced retinal neovascularization and diabetes-induced retinal vascular leakage. *Diabetes* **58**, 1902–1913 (2009).
56. De Campos, A.M., Sanchez, A., Gref, R., Calvo, P. & Alonso, M.J. The effect of a peg versus a chitosan coating on the interaction of drug colloidal carriers with the ocular mucosa. *Eur J Pharm Sci* **20**, 73–81 (2003).
57. Edelhauser, H.F., *et al.* Ophthalmic drug delivery systems for the treatment of retinal diseases: Basic research to clinical applications. *Invest Ophthalmol Vis Sci* **51**, 5403–5420 (2010).
58. Liaw, J., Chang, S.F. & Hsiao, F.C. *In vivo* gene delivery into ocular tissues by eye drops of poly(ethylene oxide)-poly(propylene oxide)-poly(efhylene oxide) (peo-ppo-peo) polymeric micelles. *Gene Thers* **8**, 999–1004 (2001).
59. Kadam, Y., Yerramilli, U., Bahadur, A. & Bahadur, P. Micelles from peo-ppo-peo block copolymers as nanocontainers for solubilization of a poorly water soluble drug hydrochlorothiazide. *Colloids Surf B Biointerfaces* **83**, 49–57 (2011).
60. Yang, C., *et al.* Intravitreal administration of dexamethasone-loaded plga-tpgs nanoparticles for the treatment of posterior segment diseases. *J Biomed Nanotechnol* **9**, 1617–1623 (2013).
61. Roy, S., *et al.* Reduction of fibronectin expression by intravitreal administration of antisense oligonucleotides. *Nat Biotechnol* **17**, 476–479 (1999).
62. Qu, X., *et al.* Carbohydrate-based micelle clusters which enhance hydrophobic drug bioavailability by up to 1 order of magnitude. *Biomacromolecules* **7**, 3452–3459 (2006).
63. Gupta, A.K., Madan, S., Majumdar, D.K. & Maitra, A. Ketorolac entrapped in polymeric micelles: Preparation, characterisation and ocular anti-inflammatory studies. *Int J Pharm* **209**, 1–14 (2000).
64. Wijagkanalan, W., Kawakami, S. & Hashida, M. Designing dendrimers for drug delivery and imaging: Pharmacokinetic considerations. *Pharm Res* **28**, 1500–1519 (2011).
65. Guzman-Aranguez, A. & Argueeso, P. Structure and biological roles of mucin-type o-glycans at the ocular surface. *Ocul Surf* **8**, 8–17 (2010).

66. Bravo-Osuna, I., *et al.* Interfacial interaction between transmembrane ocular mucins and adhesive polymers and dendrimers analyzed by surface plasmon resonance. *Pharm Res* **29**, 2329–2340 (2012).
67. Kambhampati, S.P. & Kannan, R.M. Dendrimer nanoparticles for ocular drug delivery. *J Ocul Pharmacol Ther* **29**, 151–165 (2013).
68. Shaunak, S., *et al.* Polyvalent dendrimer glucosamine conjugates prevent scar tissue formation. *Nat Biotechnol* **22**, 977–984 (2004).
69. Vandamme, T.F. & Brobeck, L. Poly(amidoamine) dendrimers as ophthalmic vehicles for ocular delivery of pilocarpine nitrate and tropicamide. *J Control Release* **102**, 23–38 (2005).
70. Zimmer, A., Mutschler, E., Lambrecht, G., Mayer, D. & Kreuter, J. Pharmacokinetic and pharmacodynamic aspects of an ophthalmic pilocarpine nanoparticle-delivery-system. *Pharm Res* **11**, 1435–1442 (1994).
71. Yang, H., Tyagi, P., Kadam, R.S., Holden, C.A. & Kompella, U.B. Hybrid dendrimer hydrogel/plga nanoparticle platform sustains drug delivery for one week and antiglaucoma effects for four days following one-time topical administration. *ACS Nano* **6**, 7595–7606 (2012).
72. Holden, C.A., *et al.* Polyamidoamine dendrimer hydrogel for enhanced delivery of antiglaucoma drugs. *Nanomed-Nanotechn Biol Med* **8**, 776–783 (2012).
73. Wang, B., *et al.* Inhibition of bacterial growth and intramniotic infection in a guinea pig model of chorioamnionitis using pamam dendrimers. *Int J Pharm* **395**, 298–308 (2010).
74. Lopez, A.I., Reins, R.Y., McDermott, A.M., Trautner, B.W. & Cai, C. Antibacterial activity and cytotoxicity of pegylated poly(amidoamine) dendrimers. *Mol BioSyst* **5**, 1148–1156 (2009).
75. Calabretta, M.K., Kumar, A., McDermott, A.M. & Cai, C. Antibacterial activities of poly(amidoamine) dendrimers terminated with amino and poly(ethylene glycol) groups. *Biomacromolecules* **8**, 1807–1811 (2007).
76. Cheng, Y., *et al.* Polyamidoamine (pamam) dendrimers as biocompatible carriers of quinolone antimicrobials: An *in vitro* study. *Eur J Med Chem* **42**, 1032–1038 (2007).
77. Grinstaff, M.W. Designing hydrogel adhesives for corneal wound repair. *Biomaterials* **28**, 5205–5214 (2007).
78. Degoricija, L., Johnson, C.S., Wathier, M., Kim, T. & Grinstaff, M.W. Photo cross-linkable biodendrimers as ophthalmic adhesives for central lacerations and penetrating keratoplasties. *Invest Ophthalmol Vis Sci* **48**, 2037–2042 (2007).

79. Berdahl, J.P., Johnson, C.S., Proia, A.D., Grinstaff, M.W. & Kim, T. Comparison of sutures and dendritic polymer adhesives for corneal laceration repair in an *in vivo* chicken model. *Arch Ophthalmol* **127**, 442–447 (2009).

80. Iezzi, R., *et al.* Dendrimer-based targeted intravitreal therapy for sustained attenuation of neuroinflammation in retinal degeneration. *Biomaterials* **33**, 979–988 (2012).

81. Kang, S.J., Durairaj, C., Kompella, U.B., O'Brien, J.M. & Grossniklaus, H.E. Subconjunctival nanoparticle carboplatin in the treatment of murine retinoblastoma. *Arch Ophthalmol* **127**, 1043–1047 (2009).

82. Makky, A., Michel, J.P., Maillard, P. & Rosilio, V. Biomimetic liposomes and planar supported bilayers for the assessment of glycodendrimeric porphyrins interaction with an immobilized lectin. *Biochim Biophys Acta Biomembr* **1808**, 656–666 (2011).

83. Timko, B.P., *et al.* Advances in drug delivery. *Annu Rev Mater Res* **41**, 1–20 (2011).

84. Kang, H.M., DeLong, R., Fisher, M.H. & Juliano, R.L. Tat-conjugated pamam dendrimers as delivery agents for antisense and sirna oligonucleotides. *Pharm Res* **22**, 2099–2106 (2005).

85. Nishiyama, N., *et al.* Light-induced gene transfer from packaged DNA enveloped in a dendrimeric photosensitizer. *Nat Mater* **4**, 934–941 (2005).

86. Raju, H.B., Hu, Y., Vedula, A., Dubovy, S.R. & Goldberg, J.L. Evaluation of magnetic micro- and nanoparticle toxicity to ocular tissues. *PLoS One* **6**, (2011).

87. Giljohann, D.A., *et al.* Gold nanoparticles for biology and medicine. *Angew Chem Int Ed* **49**, 3280–3294 (2010).

88. Dreaden, E.C., Alkilany, A.M., Huang, X., Murphy, C.J. & El-Sayed, M.A. The golden age: Gold nanoparticles for biomedicine. *Chem Soc Rev* **41**, 2740–2779 (2012).

89. Kim, J.H., *et al.* The inhibition of retinal neovascularization by gold nanoparticles via suppression of vegfr-2 activation. *Biomaterials* **32**, 1865–1871 (2011).

90. Karthikeyan, B., *et al.* Gold nanoparticles downregulate vegf-and il-1 beta-induced cell proliferation through src kinase in retinal pigment epithelial cells. *Exp Eye Res* **91**, 769–778 (2010).

91. Kalishwaralal, K., *et al.* Silver nanoparticles inhibit vegf induced cell proliferation and migration in bovine retinal endothelial cells. *Colloids Surf B* **73**, 51–57 (2009).

92. Kalishwaralal, K., BarathManiKanth, S., Pandian, S.R.K., Deepak, V. & Gurunathan, S. Silver nano — a trove for retinal therapies. *J Control Release* **145**, 76–90 (2010).

93. Jo, D.H., Kim, J.H., Yu, Y.S., Lee, T.G. & Kim, J.H. Antiangiogenic effect of silicate nanoparticle on retinal neovascularization induced by vascular endothelial growth factor. *Nanomed-Nanotechn Biol Med* **8**, 784–791 (2012).

94. Ngwa, W., Makrigiorgos, G.M. & Berbeco, R.I. Gold nanoparticle enhancement of stereotactic radiosurgery for neovascular age-related macular degeneration. *Phys Med Biol.* **57**, 6371–6380 (2012).

95. Pierscionek, B.K., *et al.* Nanoceria have no genotoxic effect on human lens epithelial cells. *Nanotechnology* **21**, (2010).

96. Zhou, X., Wong, L.L., Karakoti, A.S., Seal, S. & McGinnis, J.F. Nanoceria inhibit the development and promote the regression of pathologic retinal neovascularization in the vldlr knockout mouse. *PLoS One* **6**, (2011).

Index

achromatopsia, 17
age-related macular degeneration
(AMD), 12, 14, 15, 39, 41, 42, 47,
49, 51, 52, 55, 199, 214, 215
age-related maculopathy
susceptibility 2 (ARMS2), 64–71,
75–77, 79–82, 86, 87
ankylosing spondylitis (AS), 147,
172, 175, 178
apolipoprotein E (APOE), 65, 70, 85
AREDS supplementation, 64

Bardet-Biedl syndrome (BBS), 11, 19
Behçet's disease, 146, 155, 157, 166,
172–174, 177–179, 181

central serous chorioretinopathy, 38,
44, 49
chitosan, 201–203, 206, 207
choroidal neovascularization (CNV),
36, 37, 40–42, 44, 63, 75
neovascular AMD, 39, 55
choroidal thickness, 48
choroideremia, 20
coagulation factor XIII B chain
(F13B), 69, 81
complement component 2 (C2), 69, 81
complement component 3 (C3), 65,
66, 68, 69, 73, 79–81, 87
complement factor B (CFB), 14,
65–71, 73–83, 86–88
complement factor H (CFH), 15,
64–71, 73–83, 86–88

connective tissue growth factor
(CTGF), 69, 80, 81
Crohn's disease, 166, 172, 175,
178
cystoid macular edema (CME), 156,
159, 179, 180, 182

diabetic macular edema, 47, 55
diabetic retinopathy (DR), 14, 39, 49,
52–54

epidermal growth factor (EGF), 99,
105

fibroblast growth factor receptor-2
(FGFR2), 69, 80
frizzled homolog 4 (FZD4), 70, 71,
82, 83, 86

geographic atrophy, 51
glaucoma, 208, 215
graft-versus-host disease, 118, 125

high-temperature requirement factor
H (HTRA1), 64–70, 77–79, 81, 82,
87
hypoxia inducible factor 1 (HIF1),
14

juvenile idiopathic arthritis (JIA),
147, 163, 172, 174, 177, 178, 180
juvenile rheumatoid, 175
arthritis, 166